FATTY LIVER DIET COOKBOOK

Nutritious and Delicious Recipes for Liver Health

Henry Brown

Copyright © 2023 - All rights reserved.

The content contained within this book may not be reproduced, duplicated, or transmitted without direct written permission from the author or the publisher.

Under no circumstances will any blame or legal responsibility be held against the publisher, or author, for any damages, reparation, or monetary loss due to the information contained within this book. Either directly or indirectly.

Legal Notice:

This book is copyright protected. This book is only for personal use. You cannot amend, distribute, sell, use, quote, or paraphrase any part, or the content within this book, without the consent of the author or publisher.

Disclaimer Notice:

Please note the information contained within this document is for educational and entertainment purposes only. All effort has been executed to present accurate, up-to-date, and reliable, complete information. No warranties of any kind are declared or implied. Readers acknowledge that the author is not engaging in the rendering of legal, financial, medical, or professional advice. The content within this book has been derived from various sources. Please consult a licensed professional before attempting any techniques outlined in this book.

By reading this document, the reader agrees that under no circumstances is the author responsible for any losses, direct or indirect, which are incurred as a result of the use of the information contained within this document, including, but not limited to, — errors, omissions, or inaccuracies.

Table Of Content

Introduction 1
Causes of Fatty Liver 2
DRINK AND SMOOTHIE RECIPES 8
    STRAWBERRY SHAKE 9
    SWEET SUNRISE SMOOTHIE 10
    GREEN SEA MOSS DRINK 11
    BANANA HERBAL DRINK 13
    WATERMELON, CANTALOUPE, AND MANGO SMOOTHIE 14
    BLACKBERRY AND BANANA SMOOTHIE 15
    ORANGE AND LETTUCE SMOOTHIE 16
    GREEN TEA AND LETTUCE DETOX SMOOTHIE 17
    CHAMOMILE DELIGHT SMOOTHEE 18
    HONEY DEW AND ARUGULA SMOOTHIE 19
    WATERMELON AND STRAWBERRIES DRINK 21
    SWEET GREEN DRINK 22
    BANANA SEA MOSS SMOOTHIE 23
    SMOOTHIE BOWL 24
    REFRESHING SMOOTHIE WITH NUTS 25
    CANTALOUPE SMOOTHIE TEA 26
    WATERMELON JUICE 27
    GREEN SMOOTHEE 28
BREAKFAST RECIPES 29
    LIVER DETOX SMOOTHIE 30

HIGH PROTEIN FRENCH TOAST	32
BROCCOULI SALAD	34
CLASSIC EGGS BENEDICT WITH LEMON BASIL HOLLANDAISE	36
BLUEBERRY SMOOTHIE	38
FRIED EGG AND GREENS	39
SWEET POTATO PIE SMOOTHIE BOWL	41
SWEET POTATO PIE SMOOTHIE BOWL	42
CORNMEAL PANCAKES WITH BLACK BEAN SALSA AND CILANTRO YOGURT	43
SOUTHWESTERN-STYLE BLACK BEAN BURRITOS	45
FRUIT YOGURT PARFAIT	47
PEANUT BUTTER MAPLE BANANA MUFFINS	48
LUNCH RECIPES	**50**
MIXED VEGGIES AND GRAPEFRUIT SALAD WITH DUON GRAPEFRUIT VINAIGRETTE	51
QUICK HUMMUS AND GREEK SALAD	53
QUICK PESTO CHICKEN SALAD WITH GREENS	55
CRISPY TOFU WITH VEGETABLE SALAD	56
HEALTHY SPINACH SALAD	58
ROASTED CHICKEN AND MUSHROOMS SALAD	59
CHICKPEA, BROCCOLI, AND POMEGRANATE SALAD	60
ANCHOVY, ORANGE, AND OUVE SALAD	62
VEGETABLE AND CHICKPEA SALAD	63
TABOULI WITH VEGGIES SALAD	64
HEALTHY FATTOUSH SALAD	66
VEGGIES WITH CHICKPEA SALAD	67
CHEESY SCRAMBLED EGGS WITH FRESH HERBS	69
POULTRY AND MEAT	**71**
CHICKEN AND LEMONGRASS SAUCE	72

- SESAME CHICKEN WITH BLACK RICE, BROCCOLI, AND SNAP PEAS _____ 73
- TASTY LAMB RIBS _____ 75
- SAFFRON BEEF _____ 77
- CHICKEN AND BUTTER SAUCE _____ 79
- LEMON AND GARLIC BARBECUED OCEAN TROUT WITH GREEN SALAD ___ 81
- CHICKEN AND BLACK BEANS _____ 83
- SWEET CHIPOTLE GRILLED BEEF RIBS _____ 84
- GRILLED SIRLOIN STEAK WITH SAUCE DIANE _____ 86
- RIB ROAST WITH ROASTED SHALLOTS AND GARLIC _____ 88
- BEEF MEATBALLS _____ 89
- POT ROAST _____ 91
- BEEF TRIPE POT _____ 93
- LOVELY PULLED CHICKEN EGG BITES _____ 95

FISH AND SEAFOOD _____ 97
- SHRIMP WITH GARUC _____ 98
- SABICH SANDWICH _____ 99
- SALMON WITH VEGETABLES _____ 101
- CRISPY FISH _____ 103
- MOULES MARINIERES _____ 105
- STEAMED MUSSELS WITH COCONUT-CURRY _____ 107
- TUNA NOODLE CASSEROLE _____ 108
- SAUMON BURGERS _____ 110
- SEARED SCALLOPS _____ 112
- BLACK COD _____ 113
- MISO-GLAZED SALMON _____ 114
- ARUGULA AND SWEET POTATO SALAD _____ 115
- SHRIMP CURRY _____ 117
- SALMON PASTA _____ 119

CRAB LEGS	121
CRUSTY PESTO SALMON	122
BUTTERY COD	123
SESAME TUNA STEAK	124
LEMON GARLIC SHRIMP	125
FOIL PACKET SALMON	126
VEGETABLES	127
PARSLEY ZUCCHINI AND RADISHES	128
CHERRY TOMATOES SAUTE	130
CREAMY EGGPLANT	132
EGGPLANT AND CARROTS MIX	134
PARMESAN EGGPLANTS	135
KALE SAUTE	136
CARROTS SAUTE	137
SPAGHETTI SQUASH CASSEROLE	138
SUPER TASTY ONION PETALS	140
EGGPLANT GARLIC SALAD WITH TOMATOES	142
CURRY EGGPLANTS	144
SAUTEED ASPARAGUS	146
ROASTED APPLE WITH BACON	147
FENNEL SLICES	148
BUTTERNUT SQUASH RICE	149
EGGPLANT LASAGNA	150
STUFFED EGGPLANTS WITH CHERRY TOMATOES	152
SALADS	154
SATISFYING SPRING SALAD	155
THE RAW GREEN DETOX SALAD	157
DANDELION SALAD	159

SPICY WAKAME SALAD	160
AVO-ORANGE SALAD DISH	161
NOURISHING ELECTRIC SALAD	162
SUPERFOOD FONIO SALAD	163
HEALTHY CHICKPEA ROAST SALAD	165
AMARANTH TABBOULEH SALAD	166
ZUCCHINI AND MUSHROOM BOWL	168
QUINOA, TOMATO, AND MANGO SALAD	169

Introduction

A Fatty Liver Diet cookbook is an anthology of culinary instructions and dietary advice intended to assist individuals suffering from fatty liver disease to regulate their condition through appropriate nutrition. Fatty liver disease is a disorder characterized by an excessive buildup of fat in the liver, resulting in inflammation and damage. The cookbook is crafted to offer wholesome, nutritious, and tasty food options that bolster liver health and encourage weight reduction, which can be vital elements in minimizing the likelihood of liver injury. The recipes typically include ingredients low in fat, sugar, and salt, and may also encompass guidelines for portion management and lifestyle modifications to sustain liver health.

Causes of Fatty Liver

Fatty liver disease arises when surplus fat accumulates in the liver, instigating inflammation and damage. Several prevalent causes of fatty liver encompass:

1. Alcohol overconsumption: Heavy intake of alcohol is among the leading causes of fatty liver.
2. Obesity: Excess body fat can augment the volume of fat stored in the liver.
3. Insulin resistance: Conditions like type 2 diabetes and metabolic syndrome can precipitate insulin resistance, which can then lead to fat buildup in the liver.
4. Rapid weight loss: Shedding weight too quickly can trigger the liver to discharge large quantities of stored fat into the bloodstream, resulting in fatty liver.
5. High-fat diets: Diets high in saturated and trans fats can augment the volume of fat stored in the liver.
6. Certain medications: Some drugs, such as corticosteroids, can provoke fatty liver.
7. Viral hepatitis: Inflammation due to viral hepatitis can also instigate fatty liver. It's crucial to understand that sometimes fatty liver can develop without any apparent cause. Maintaining a healthy lifestyle, eating a balanced diet, and seeking professional healthcare consultation if you have worries about your liver health are essential.

Signs and Symptoms of Fatty Liver

Fatty liver disease often remains symptomless in its initial stages. However, as the condition advances, some individuals might experience:

1. Fatigue and weakness
2. Discomfort or pain in the upper right quadrant of the abdomen
3. Weight loss
4. Nausea
5. Anomalies in liver function tests
6. Elevated liver enzymes in the bloodstream
7. High cholesterol levels
8. High blood pressure
9. Type 2 diabetes If you have any apprehensions about your liver health, it's vital to consult a healthcare professional for an appropriate evaluation. Early detection and treatment of fatty liver disease can help impede the progression to more severe liver issues.

Prevention of Fatty Liver Disease

Fatty liver disease can often be averted or reversed through lifestyle modifications and healthy practices. Some ways to prevent fatty liver disease include:

1. Maintaining a healthy weight: Weight loss, especially if you're overweight or obese, can help lessen the quantity of fat stored in the liver.
2. Adopting a healthy diet: A diet low in fat, sugar, and processed foods and high in fiber, fruits, and vegetables can help bolster liver health.

3. Regular exercise: Frequent physical activity can aid in weight loss, reduce insulin resistance, and enhance liver function.
4. Limiting alcohol intake: Heavy alcohol intake is a common cause of fatty liver, so it's crucial to limit your alcohol consumption or avoid it entirely.
5. Regulating blood sugar levels: If you're living with type 2 diabetes, it's crucial to control your blood sugar levels through diet, exercise, and medication to reduce the risk of fatty liver.
6. Managing viral hepatitis: If you have viral hepatitis, following your healthcare professional's treatment recommendations is vital to prevent further liver damage.
7. Avoiding certain medications: Some medications, like corticosteroids, can cause fatty liver, so it's essential to discuss with your doctor the risks and benefits of any medication you're taking. By implementing these changes and embracing healthy habits, you can help lower your risk of developing fatty liver disease and improve your overall liver health.

What is a Fatty Liver Diet?

A fatty liver diet is a dietary regimen aimed at aiding the management of fatty liver disease by promoting wholesome, nutritious food options. The objective of a fatty liver diet is to lessen the amount of fat stored in the liver, enhance liver function, and support overall health. This can be accomplished by focusing on low-fat, fiber-rich foods, such as fruits and vegetables, whole grains, and lean protein, and avoiding foods high in fat, sugar, and processed foods. It's important to consult a healthcare professional before starting a fatty liver diet, as individual nutritional needs vary, and a personalized diet plan is recommended.

Suggested Food Intake

For a diet that targets fatty liver disease, it is beneficial to consume foods low in fat and rich in nutrients, fiber, and protein. Here are some excellent choices for a fatty liver diet:

1. Fruits: Fresh fruits like apples, bananas, oranges, berries, among others, are full of vitamins and antioxidants, high in fiber, and low in calories.

2. Vegetables: Nutrient-rich, low-calorie leafy greens, cruciferous vegetables, and other non-starchy vegetables should be included.

3. Whole grains: Foods like whole-grain breads, cereals, pasta, and brown rice are rich in fiber and deliver sustained energy without causing drastic blood sugar fluctuations.

4. Lean protein: Low-fat sources of protein like fish, poultry, tofu, and legumes are great options and also provide essential nutrients, including omega-3 fatty acids.

5. Nuts and seeds: Healthy snacks like almonds, chia seeds, and other nuts and seeds are high in good fats, protein, and fiber.

6. Low-fat dairy: Items like low-fat milk, yogurt, and cheese are rich sources of calcium, protein, and other vital nutrients.

7. Healthy fats: Foods like olive oil, avocados, and fatty fish such as salmon are packed with beneficial monounsaturated and omega-3 fatty acids, supporting liver health.

Before making any significant changes to your diet, consulting with a healthcare professional is recommended as everyone's nutritional needs and food tolerances are different. They can assist you in creating a personalized diet plan that suits you.

Foods to Refrain From

To help manage fatty liver disease, it's crucial to avoid foods high in fat, sugar, and salt. Here are some food types to refrain from on a fatty liver diet:

1. Fried foods: Items like french fries, fried chicken, and doughnuts are laden with unhealthy fats and lead to weight gain and liver damage.
2. Processed foods: Foods like snack foods, baked goods, and pre-packaged meals often contain high levels of sugar, salt, and unhealthy fats, which can harm the liver.
3. High-fat dairy: High-fat dairy products like whole milk, cream, and cheese can contribute to weight gain and liver damage.
4. Sugary drinks: Drinks high in sugar content, such as soda, energy drinks, and fruit juice, can cause weight gain, insulin resistance, and liver damage.
5. Alcohol: Alcohol is calorically dense and can damage the liver, so limiting or avoiding alcohol is essential.
6. Red meat: Red meat is high in saturated fat, leading to weight gain and potential liver damage.
7. Sweet treats: Desserts and candies are high in sugar and unhealthy fats and should be consumed in moderation, if at all.

Again, before making any significant changes to your diet, it is important to consult a healthcare professional. They can guide you based on your specific nutritional needs and food tolerances and assist in creating a personalized diet plan that suits you.

DRINK AND SMOOTHIE RECIPES

STRAWBERRY SHAKE

Cook Time: 5 minutes

Serving: 4 servings

Ingredients:

- 3 cups of fresh strawberries, diced
- 1/2 cup granulated sugar
- 2 cups of heavy cream
- 2 teaspoons of vanilla extract

Preparation:

1. In a blender, add the diced strawberries and sugar and blend until smooth. Set aside.
2. In a bowl, whip the heavy cream until stiff peaks form.
3. Add the strawberry mixture to the whipped cream and stir together until fully combined.
4. Add in the vanilla extract and mix again until fully incorporated into the shake.
5. Divide the shake among four glasses or mason jars and enjoy!

Nutrition:

Each serving of Strawberry Shake contains approximately 545 calories, 25g of fat, 77g of carbohydrates, and 4g of protein. Enjoy!

SWEET SUNRISE SMOOTHIE

Cook Time: 5 minutes

Serving: 1 smoothie

Ingredients:

- 1/2 cup frozen mango cubes
- 1 banana, cut into chunks
- 1 teaspoon honey
- 1/2 cup plain Greek yogurt
- 1/2 cup orange juice or pineapple juice
- A few ice cubes (optional)

Preparation:

1. Place the frozen mango cubes in a blender and blend until they are mostly smooth.
2. Add the banana chunks, honey, yogurt and orange juice to the blender and blend until it is thick and creamy. If necessary, add some ice cubes to thicken it up.
3. Pour the smoothie into a glass and enjoy!

Nutrition:

One serving of this smoothie provides 349 calories, 5g fat, 1g saturated fat, 0mg cholesterol, 37g carbohydrates, 32g sugar, 10g protein and 4g fiber. It also contains 128% of the daily recommended intake of vitamin C. Enjoy!

GREEN SEA MOSS DRINK

Cook Time: 10 minutes

Servings: 1-2

Ingredients:

- 2 cups of boiling water
- ½ cup green sea moss
- 2-4 tablespoons of maple syrup or honey (optional)
- Your favorite fruit juice or smoothie base for additional flavor (optional)

Preparation:

1. Put the green sea moss in a bowl, and pour the boiling water over it. Let sit for 15 minutes to soften.
2. Once softened, rinse and strain the sea moss several times to remove any impurities. Place it in a blender with enough filtered water to cover it completely. Blend on high speed until the mixture is smooth and creamy - about 1 minute.
3. If you would like a sweeter taste, add 2-4 tablespoons of maple syrup or honey to the blender. Also add any additional flavor of your choice - such as a splash of fruit juice or smoothie base - and blend until combined.
4. Pour the mixture into glasses and serve cold with ice cubes if desired.

Nutrition:

Green sea moss is an incredibly nutritious food that contains plenty of vitamins, minerals and other beneficial compounds. It is rich in iodine, calcium, magnesium, zinc and potassium, as well as antioxidants and anti-inflammatory compounds that can help support optimal health. Additionally, it may aid digestion, boost immunity and even reduce stress levels! Enjoy this delicious green sea moss drink to reap all its health benefits!

BANANA HERBAL DRINK

Cook time: 5 minutes

Serving: 2 servings

Ingredients:

- 2 bananas, cut into small pieces
- 1 cup of herbal tea (such as chamomile or ginger)
- Honey to taste Ice cubes (optional)

Preparation:

1. Put the banana pieces and ice cubes in a blender and blend for about 30 seconds until smooth.
2. Pour the blended mixture into two glasses and add one cup of herbal tea to each glass.
3. Add honey to taste and stir thoroughly.
4. Serve chilled or with extra ice cubes if desired.

Nutrition:

This recipe provides approximately 85 calories per serving, along with essential vitamins and minerals. The herbal tea provides antioxidants which can help reduce inflammation and boost immunity. Honey is a good source of energy, as well as being rich in various vitamins and minerals. The banana provides dietary fiber and potassium, both important for healthy digestion. Enjoy!

WATERMELON, CANTALOUPE, AND MANGO SMOOTHIE

Cook Time: 10 minutes

Servings: 2 people

Ingredients:

- ½ cup (80 g) of diced watermelon
- ½ cup (75 g) of diced cantaloupe
- ½ cup (100 g) of diced mango
- 1 tablespoon honey or agave nectar for sweetness, optional

Preparation:

1. Place the diced fruits in a blender and blend until creamy.
2. If needed, add in some honey or agave nectar to sweeten the smoothie.
3. Pour into two glasses and enjoy!

Nutrition Information:

Calories 135; Total Fat 0g; Sodium 9mg; Potassium 447 mg; Total Carbs 34g; Dietary Fiber 2.3g; Sugars 28.5g; Protein 1.9g. Enjoy!

BLACKBERRY AND BANANA SMOOTHIE

Cook time: 5 minutes

Serving: 2 smoothies

Ingredients:
- 1 banana, peeled and sliced
- 1 cup of blackberries, fresh or frozen
- 1 tablespoon honey
- ½ cup of milk (or dairy free alternative)
- Ice cubes, optional

Preparation:
1. Place all the ingredients in a blender.
2. Blend until you get a creamy and homogeneous mixture.
3. Pour into two glasses and enjoy!

Nutrition information:

Calories – 131 kcal Carbohydrates – 30 g Protein – 3 g Fat – 2 g Fiber – 4 g Sugar – 20 g Sodium – 18 mg.

ORANGE AND LETTUCE SMOOTHIE

Cook time: 10 minutes

Servings: 2

Ingredients:

- 1/2 cup orange juice, freshly squeezed
- 1/4 of a head of lettuce, chopped into small pieces
- 2 tablespoons honey
- 1 teaspoon vanilla extract
- 2 cups ice cubes (optional)

Preparation:

1. Place orange juice, lettuce, honey, and vanilla extract in a blender or food processor. Blend until smooth.
2. Add the ice cubes if desired and blend again for 30 seconds or until the mixture is completely combined and smooth.
3. Pour into two glasses and serve immediately. Enjoy!

Nutrition:

Each serving contains approximately 201 calories, 0.8 g fat, 49.7 g carbohydrates, and 2.6 g protein. This smoothie is also a good source of vitamins A and C as well as fiber. It can be a great addition to any breakfast or snack! Happy blending!

GREEN TEA AND LETTUCE DETOX SMOOTHIE

Cook time: 5 minutes

Serving: 2 servings

Ingredients:

- 1 cup green tea, cold
- 2 cups of fresh lettuce, chopped
- 1 banana, sliced
- ½ cup frozen pineapple cubes, or mango if preferred
- ¾ cup almond milk or other plant-based milk of choice

Preparation:

1. In a blender place the green tea, lettuce and banana; blend until smooth. Add in the pineapple and almond milk; blend until all ingredients are combined. Serve immediately and enjoy!

Nutrition

(per serving): Calories: 86 kcal; Carbs: 17g; Fat: 2g; Protein: 3g.

This smoothie is a great way to get in some greens and detoxify your body. Enjoy!

CHAMOMILE DELIGHT SMOOTHEE

Cook Time: 15 minutes

Serving Size: 2-3 servings

Ingredients:

- 1 banana, peeled and cut into chunks
- 2 cups of frozen chamomile tea leaves
- 1/4 cup honey or agave nectar
- 1 cup plain Greek yogurt
- 2 tablespoons freshly squeezed lemon juice
- 1 teaspoon ground ginger

Preparation:

2. In a blender, combine the banana and tea leaves. Blend for about 1 minute until smooth. Add the honey or agave nectar, yogurt, lemon juice and ground ginger. Blend for another 30 seconds until creamy.
3. Serve immediately in glasses topped with fresh fruit if desired. Enjoy!

Nutrition:

Serving Size- 1 cup. Calories- 182, Fat- 2g, Carbohydrates- 38g, Protein -7g. This recipe is high in fiber and vitamin C. It's also a great source of calcium and iron! Enjoy!

HONEY DEW AND ARUGULA SMOOTHIE

Cook time: 8 minutes.

Servings: 2.

Ingredients:

- 1 cup honeydew melon, cubed
- 1 cup arugula leaves, washed and dried
- ½ cup ice cubes
- ¼ cup almond milk or other plant-based milk of choice
- 1 tablespoon fresh lemon juice

Preparation:

1. Place the honeydew melon in a blender and blend until smooth.
2. Add the arugula leaves and blend until smooth.
3. Add the ice cubes, almond milk, and lemon juice and blend again until fully combined and creamy.
4. Serve immediately in two glasses or store in an airtight container in the refrigerator for up to two days.

Nutrition:

One serving of this smoothie contains 130 calories, 2 grams of fat, 26 grams of carbohydrates, 6 grams of protein, and 3 grams of dietary fiber. It is also a good source of vitamins A, C, K, and several other essential nutrients. The honeydew melon provides a sweet flavor while the arugula leaves provide a slightly bitter taste that helps balance out the sweetness. Enjoy this flavorful and refreshing smoothie as a healthy snack or part of your breakfast!

WATERMELON AND STRAWBERRIES DRINK

Cook Time: 10 minutes

Serving: Makes 8 servings

Ingredients:

- 4 cups seedless watermelon, diced
- 2 cups fresh strawberries, sliced
- 2 tablespoons honey (optional)
- 2 tablespoons freshly squeezed lime juice
- 1/2 teaspoon freshly grated ginger (optional)

Preparation:

1. In a blender, combine the diced watermelon, fresh strawberries, honey (if desired), lime juice and ginger (if desired). Blend until smooth. Taste and adjust sweetness, if necessary.
2. Pour the mixture into a large pitcher or container and refrigerate for 1 hour before serving.
3. Serve over ice with extra lime wedges and fresh mint leaves (optional).

Nutrition:

Per serving: Calories 41, Total Fat 0g, Sodium 8mg, Potassium 183mg, Protein 1g, Carbohydrate 10g, Fiber 2g.

SWEET GREEN DRINK

Cook Time: 5 minutes

Serving Size: 2-3 glasses

Ingredients:

- 1 banana
- 1 kiwi (peeled)
- ½ cup pineapple juice
- 2 cups kale or spinach leaves
- 1 teaspoon honey (optional)

Preparation:

1. In a blender, combine the banana, kiwi, pineapple juice and kale/spinach leaves. Blend until smooth.
2. Pour into glasses and add a teaspoon of honey to each, if desired.

Nutrition:

Each serving contains approximately 150 calories and is packed with essential vitamins and minerals like vitamin C, folate, iron and calcium. Enjoy!

BANANA SEA MOSS SMOOTHIE

Cook Time: 10 minutes

Serving: 2-4 people

Ingredients:

- 1 ripe banana
- 2 tablespoons of Sea Moss Gel powder
- 1 cup of orange juice
- ½ teaspoon of vanilla extract (optional)

Preparation:

1. Peel the banana and place the pieces into a blender.
2. Add sea moss gel, orange juice, and vanilla extract to the blender. Blend until all ingredients are well incorporated and smooth.
3. Pour mixture into glasses and serve chilled or at room temperature. Enjoy!

Nutrition Information

(Based on 4 servings): Calories – 108, Total Fat – 0g, Saturated fat – 0g, Cholesterol – 0mg, Sodium – 5mg, Carbohydrate – 27g, Dietary Fiber – 2g, Protein – 1.5g.

SMOOTHIE BOWL

Cook Time: 5 minutes

Serving: 1 bowl

Ingredients:

- 1/2 cup frozen mango chunks
- 1/2 banana, frozen and sliced
- 1/4 cup non-dairy milk of choice (such as almond or coconut)
- 2 tablespoons hemp seeds
- Optional toppings of your choice such as granola, fresh fruit, nut butter, and chia seeds

Preparation:

1. Place the mango chunks and banana slices into a food processor or blender. Pulse until everything is broken down into small pieces.
2. Add in the non-dairy milk and blend on high for about 2 minutes until the smoothie is thick and creamy.
3. Pour into a bowl and top with hemp seeds and your desired toppings.

Nutrition:

Calories: 250; Total Fat: 8g; Saturated Fat: 1g; Sodium: 5mg; Carbohydrates: 37g; Fiber: 6g; Protein: 10g.

REFRESHING SMOOTHIE WITH NUTS

Cook Time: 2 minutes

Servings: 1

Ingredients:

- 1 cup frozen mango chunks
- 1/2 cup plain yogurt
- 1 tablespoon chia seeds soaked in
- 1/3 cup water, or almond milk
- 1/4 teaspoon ground cardamom
- 2 tablespoons honey or agave nectar
- 2 tablespoons of crushed nuts (almonds, walnuts, or cashews)

Preparation:

1. Combine all ingredients in a blender and blend until it is smooth. Make sure to blend for at least 1-2 minutes to ensure all ingredients are properly blended.

Nutrition (per serving):

Calories: 330, Protein: 9g, Fat: 10g, Carbs: 51g, Fiber: 6g, Sugar: 37g. Enjoy!

CANTALOUPE SMOOTHIE TEA

Cook Time: 5 minutes

Servings: 1-2

Ingredients:

- 1 cup of cantaloupe
- 1/4 cup of freshly brewed tea (you can use any type you like)
- 1 tablespoon of honey or sugar for sweetness
- Ice cubes as desired (optional)

Preparation:

2. Start by cutting the cantaloupe into small cubes (about 1 inch each). Place the cubes into a blender.
3. Add the freshly brewed tea and sweetener to the blender.
4. Blend until smooth.
5. Transfer the liquid into glasses and add in desired amount of ice cubes (optional).
6. Serve immediately and enjoy!

Nutrition:

One serving of this Cantaloupe Smoothie Tea contains approximately 105 calories, 24 grams of carbohydrates, 2 grams of protein and 0 fat. It is a great source of Vitamin A, C and potassium as well as other essential vitamins and minerals. Enjoy!

WATERMELON JUICE

Cook Time: 15 minutes

Serving: 4 glasses

Ingredients:

- 4 cups of watermelon, cubed
- 1/2 cup fresh lime juice
- 3 tablespoons sugar (more or less to taste)
- Ice cubes (optional)

Preparation:

1. Place the cubed watermelon in a blender and blend until smooth. Strain the mixture through a fine mesh sieve into a bowl or pitcher and discard any remaining solids.
2. Add the lime juice and sugar to the puree and stir until dissolved. Taste and adjust accordingly with additional sugar if needed.
3. For a cold beverage, add ice cubes to each glass before pouring the watermelon juice.
4. Serve and enjoy!

Nutrition:

Calories: 64 kcal, Carbohydrates: 16 g, Protein: 1 g, Fat: 0 g, Saturated Fat: 0 g, Sodium: 4 mg, Potassium: 191 mg, Fiber: 1g, Sugar: 13 g Vitamin A 12%, Vitamin C 28% Calcium 2%, Iron 3%.

GREEN SMOOTHEE

Cook Time: 10 minutes

Servings: 2 servings

Ingredients:

- 1 cup of spinach
- 2 ripe bananas, peeled and chopped
- 1/2 cup almond milk
- 3 tablespoons honey or agave nectar (optional)
- 2 teaspoons ground cinnamon
- ½ teaspoon ground nutmeg
- Optional - handful of ice cubes for a thicker smoothie

Preparation:

1. Place the spinach in a blender and blend until it's finely chopped. Add the rest of the ingredients to the blender and blend on high speed until you reach your desired consistency. You may need to add more liquid if the mixture is too thick.
2. Pour into two glasses and serve.

Nutrition:

One serving provides approximately 263 calories, 6 g of protein, 53 g of carbohydrates and 5 g fat. It also contains a significant amount of fiber and vitamins A, C, K and B-6. Enjoy!

BREAKFAST RECIPES

LIVER DETOX SMOOTHIE

Cook Time: 10 minutes

Servings: 1-2 people

Ingredients:

- ½ cup frozen pineapple chunks
- ½ cup fresh spinach leaves
- 1 medium cucumber, chopped
- 1 small orange, peeled and quartered
- 2 tablespoons freshly squeezed lemon juice
- 1 teaspoon chia seeds
- 1 teaspoon ground ginger
- 2 cups purified water or unsweetened nut milk of your choice (almond, oat, hemp)

Preparation:

1. Combine all ingredients together in a blender and blend until smooth. Add more liquid if needed to reach desired consistency.
2. Serve immediately or store in the refrigerator for up to 3 days.

Nutrition Information:

For every 8-ounce serving, this smoothie contains approximately 165 calories, with 6 grams of protein, 2.5g fat and 27 grams of carbs. The fiber content is 3 grams per serving and the sugar content is 12 grams per serving. This smoothie also provides 1 gram of iron per serving and 20% Vitamin C of your recommended daily intake (RDI). It's a great way to start your day or have as an afternoon snack! Enjoy!

HIGH PROTEIN FRENCH TOAST

Cook Time: 10 minutes

Servings: 2

Ingredients:

- 4 slices of bread
- 2 eggs
- 1/4 cup milk
- 1 tsp cinnamon
- 1 tbsp maple syrup or honey (optional)
- 1 scoop of protein powder (optional)

Preparation:

1. Preheat the skillet over medium heat. Grease it with a little bit of butter or oil.
2. Crack two eggs into a bowl and whisk them together vigorously with the milk and optional protein powder until it's completely mixed together. Then add in the cinnamon and optional sweetener, mixing to combine everything together well.
3. Dip each side of your bread into the egg mixture, making sure it's fully coated.
4. Place the bread onto your preheated skillet and cook until golden brown on each side (about 2-3 minutes per side).
5. Serve with a drizzle of honey or syrup, if desired. Enjoy!

Nutrition:

Calories: 227 | Fat: 5 g | Carbs: 25 g | Protein: 13 g

BROCCOULI SALAD

Cook time: 15-20 minutes

Serving: 4 servings

Ingredients:

- 2 heads of broccoli, cut into florets
- 1/2 cup olive oil
- Juice of 1/2 lemon
- 2 cloves garlic, minced
- Salt and pepper to taste
- 2 tablespoons Parmesan cheese, grated or shredded
- 2 tablespoons pine nuts (optional)

Preparation:

1. Preheat the oven to 375°F. Line a baking sheet with parchment paper.
2. Place the broccoli florets on the prepared baking sheet and drizzle with the olive oil, lemon juice, and garlic. Toss gently to combine and season with salt and pepper.
3. Roast in the preheated oven for 15-20 minutes, or until tender and golden brown.
4. Remove from the oven and top with Parmesan cheese and pine nuts (if using). Serve immediately.

Nutrition:

Serving Size: 1/4 of recipe • Calories: 160 • Fat: 13g • Carbs: 8g • Protein: 4g • Fiber: 3g • Sugar: 2g Sodium: 124mg (without added salt) *Nutritional information is an estimate and not guaranteed to be accurate. Please consult a registered dietician for special diets or specific needs.

CLASSIC EGGS BENEDICT WITH LEMON BASIL HOLLANDAISE

Cook Time: 25 minutes

Serving: 4 servings

Ingredients:

- 2 English muffins, halved & toasted
- 8 slices of cooked ham or Canadian bacon
- 2 tablespoons butter, melted
- 8 large eggs

Preparation:

1. Preheat oven to 425°F (220°C). Grease a baking sheet with butter or nonstick cooking spray and set aside.

2. Place the English muffins, cut side up, on prepared baking sheet. Top each half with one slice of ham or Canadian bacon and brush lightly with melted butter.

3. Bake in preheated oven until warmed through, about 5 minutes. Remove from oven and keep warm while preparing Hollandaise sauce and poached eggs.

4. To prepare the Hollandaise sauce, whisk together egg yolks, lemon juice, mustard, cayenne pepper (if using), and salt in a medium heat-proof bowl. Set over a pan of barely simmering water and whisk constantly until mixture is thickened and doubled in volume, about 3 minutes.

5. Remove from heat and gradually whisk in melted butter, a few tablespoons at a time, until sauce has reached desired

consistency. Stir in basil. Adjust seasoning with additional salt if necessary.

6. To poach eggs, fill a large skillet halfway with water and bring to a gentle simmer. Crack each egg into its own cup or ramekin then slide gently into the simmering water. Poach for 3 minutes or until whites are set but yolks are still runny (longer if desired). Gently remove eggs with slotted spoon and set aside.

7. To assemble the Eggs Benedict, place two muffin halves on each plate and top with two poached eggs. Drizzle with Hollandaise sauce and serve immediately.

Nutrition:

Calories 489; Fat 34 g; Cholesterol 355 mg; Sodium 837 mg; Carbohydrates 22 g; Fiber 2 g; Protein 23 g.

BLUEBERRY SMOOTHIE

Cook Time: 15 minutes

Serving: Makes 1 large smoothie

Ingredients:

- ½ cup blueberries, fresh or frozen
- ½ banana, frozen
- ¾ cup plain yogurt
- 2 tablespoons honey (or to taste)
- ⅓ cup almond milk (or other dairy/non-dairy milk of choice)

Preparation:

1. Place all ingredients in the blender and blend until smooth.
2. Serve immediately or store in an airtight container in the refrigerator for up to 48 hours.

Nutrition:

Calories – 286, Fat – 4g, Protein – 9g, Carbohydrates – 54g, Sugar – 36g, Fiber – 4g. Enjoy your freshly made blueberry smoothie!

FRIED EGG AND GREENS

Cook Time: 15 minutes

Servings: 4

Ingredients:

- 1 tablespoon olive oil
- 2 cloves garlic, minced
- 4 large eggs
- Salt and pepper to taste
- 3 cups of fresh chopped kale or spinach
- ¼ teaspoon cayenne pepper (optional)

Preparation:

1. Heat the oil in a medium skillet over medium heat. Add the garlic and cook for 1 minute until fragrant.
2. Crack the eggs into the pan and season with salt & pepper. Cook for about 5 minutes until whites are set but yolks remain soft; cover if desired to help speed up cooking time.
3. Add the kale or spinach and cayenne pepper, stirring to combine. Cook for an additional 2-3 minutes until the greens are wilted.
4. Serve with your favorite toast or breakfast side dish, and enjoy!

Nutrition:

Serving size 1/4 of recipe; Calories 166; Total fat 10 g; Saturated fat 3 g; Cholesterol 186 mg; Sodium 114 mg; Potassium 367 mg;

Total carbohydrates 6 g; Dietary fiber 2 g ; Sugars 0 g ; Protein 12g.

SWEET POTATO PIE SMOOTHIE BOWL

Cook time: 10 minutes

Serving: 1 bowl

Ingredients:

- 1/2 cup cooked, mashed sweet potato
- 1 banana, sliced and frozen
- 1/4 cup almond milk
- 1 scoop of your favorite vanilla protein powder
- 1 teaspoon cinnamon
- Pinch of nutmeg

Preparation:

1. In a blender, blend the mashed sweet potato, banana slices, and almond milk until smooth.
2. Add the protein powder, cinnamon, and nutmeg to the blender and pulse a few times to combine.
3. Pour the mixture into a bowl and top with desired toppings like chopped nuts or shredded coconut. Enjoy!

Nutrition:

Serving Size 1 bowl | Calories 310, Total Fat 8g, Saturated Fat 2g, Trans Fat 0g, Cholesterol 0mg, Sodium 315mg, Total Carbohydrate 34g, Dietary Fiber 6g, Sugars 13.5g, Protein 21.5g.

SWEET POTATO PIE SMOOTHIE BOWL

Cook Time: 15 minutes

Servings: 4 servings

Ingredients:

- 2 cooked sweet potatoes, peeled and mashed
- 2 Bananas
- 1/2 cup Almond Milk
- 2 tablespoons Maple Syrup
- 1 teaspoon Vanilla Extract
- 1/4 teaspoon Cinnamon

Preparation:

1. In a blender, combine the mashed sweet potatoes, bananas, almond milk, maple syrup, vanilla extract and cinnamon. Blend until smooth.
2. Pour the smoothie into four bowls and top with desired toppings (chopped nuts, chia seeds, coconut flakes etc.). Enjoy!

Nutrition Information per Serving:

Calories 160; Fat 0g; Cholesterol 0mg; Sodium 11mg; Carbohydrate 37g; Fiber 4g; Sugar 17g; Protein 2g.

CORNMEAL PANCAKES WITH BLACK BEAN SALSA AND CILANTRO YOGURT

Cook time: 30 minutes

Serving: 4 servings

Ingredients:

- 1 cup cornmeal
- 1 teaspoon baking powder
- 1/2 teaspoon salt
- 2 tablespoons honey
- 2 eggs, beaten
- 2 cups milk (or unsweetened almond milk)
- 2 tablespoons olive oil or butter, melted, plus more for cooking pancakes

For the salsa:

- 1 can black beans, drained and rinsed
- 1/2 red onion, diced
- 1 bell pepper, diced (any color will do!)
- 2 tablespoons lime juice

For the cilantro yogurt:

- 1 cup plain Greek yogurt
- 2 tablespoons fresh cilantro, chopped
- 1 teaspoon honey

Preparation:

1. In a large bowl, whisk together the cornmeal, baking powder and salt. Stir in the honey, eggs, milk and melted oil or butter until combined. Let sit for 5 minutes to allow the batter to thicken up.
2. Heat a griddle over medium heat and lightly grease with cooking spray or oil of choice. Scoop about ¼ cup of pancake batter onto the griddle and cook for 2-3 minutes per side until golden brown. Repeat with remaining pancakes - you should get around 10 pancakes total!
3. For the salsa; in a medium bowl, combine the black beans, onion, bell pepper and lime juice. Mix until evenly combined.
4. For the cilantro yogurt; in a small bowl whisk together yogurt, cilantro and honey until creamy and smooth.
5. Serve pancakes topped with black bean salsa and a dollop of cilantro yogurt! Enjoy!

Nutrition:

Calories: 287kcal | Carbohydrates: 44g | Protein: 10g | Fat: 7g | Saturated Fat: 2g | Cholesterol: 64mg | Sodium: 335mg | Potassium: 320mg | Fiber: 5g Sugar 11g Vitamin A :

645IU| Vitamin C : 24mg| Calcium: 185mg| Iron: 2.3mg

SOUTHWESTERN-STYLE BLACK BEAN BURRITOS

Cook Time: 20 minutes

Serving: 4 Servings

Ingredients:

- 2 Tablespoons olive oil
- 1 medium onion, diced
- 1 red bell pepper, diced
- 1 jalapeño, seeded and minced (optional)
- 2 cloves garlic, minced
- 1 teaspoon ground cumin
- ¼ teaspoon chili powder (or to taste)
- ½ teaspoon salt (or to taste)
- 2 cans black beans, drained and rinsed
- 8 large flour tortillas

Preparation:

1. Heat the oil in a large skillet over medium heat.
2. Add the onion, bell pepper, jalapeño (if using), and garlic. Sauté for about 5 minutes until vegetables are softened.
3. Stir in the cumin, chili powder, salt and black beans. Cook for another 5 minutes to allow flavors to combine.
4. Warm each of the 8 tortillas according to package instructions. Place 1/4 cup of the black bean mixture onto each one, fold up

into a burrito shape and serve with your favorite toppings like salsa or guacamole!

Nutrition:

Each serving of this Black Bean Burrito has approximately 320 calories, 65g of carbohydrates and 10g of protein! It is also a good source of dietary fiber, vitamin C and iron. Enjoy!

FRUIT YOGURT PARFAIT

Cook Time: 15 minutes

Servings: 4

Ingredients:

- 2 cups plain Greek yogurt
- 1 cup fresh berries (or other seasonal fruit)
- 2 tablespoons honey or agave syrup, optional
- ¼ cup almonds, chopped
- ¼ cup granola of your choice

Preparation:

1. In a medium bowl mix together the yogurt and honey or agave syrup until well combined. Taste and adjust sweetness as desired.
2. Layer into four glasses or bowls the yogurt, berries, almonds and granola in that order. With each layer, press down slightly to compact it before adding the next layer. Repeat until finished with all ingredients.
3. Serve immediately or chill until ready to serve. Enjoy!

Nutrition:

Per Serving: Calories 181, Protein 12 g (24%), Carbohydrate 15 g (30%), Total Fat 8 g (46%), Fiber 3 g, Vitamin A 2%, Vitamin C 19%, Calcium 20%, Iron 8%.

PEANUT BUTTER MAPLE BANANA MUFFINS

Cook time: 25 minutes

Serving: 10 muffins

Ingredients:

- ½ cup creamy peanut butter
- ¼ cup maple syrup
- 1 ripe banana, mashed
- 2 eggs
- 1 cup all-purpose flour
- ½ teaspoon baking soda

Preparation:

1. Preheat oven to 375°F. Grease a standard size muffin tin with nonstick cooking spray or line with paper liners.
2. In a medium bowl, combine the peanut butter and maple syrup until smooth and creamy.
3. Stir in the mashed banana and eggs until combined.
4. Add the flour and baking soda, stirring just until no dry spots remain.
5. Divide the batter evenly among the 10 muffin cups, filling each about two-thirds full.
6. Bake for 25 minutes or until a toothpick inserted in the center comes out clean. Let cool slightly before serving.

Nutrition Information:

Calories per muffin – 181; Fat – 7g; Carbohydrates – 24g; Protein – 6g; Fiber - 2g; Cholesterol - 33mg.

LUNCH RECIPES

MIXED VEGGIES AND GRAPEFRUIT SALAD WITH DUON GRAPEFRUIT VINAIGRETTE

Cook Time: 10 minutes

Servings: 4-6

Ingredients:

- 2 grapefruits, peeled and divided into segments
- 2 cups mixed vegetables (carrots, bell peppers, cauliflower, broccoli)
- ¼ cup olive oil
- 2 tablespoons white wine vinegar or lemon juice
- 1 teaspoon honey or sugar
- Salt and pepper to taste

Preparation:

1. Begin by preparing the vegetables for the salad - wash them thoroughly and cut into bitesized pieces. Set aside in a large bowl.
2. Prepare the dressing by combining the olive oil, white wine vinegar or lemon juice, honey or sugar, salt and pepper in a small bowl and whisk until blended.
3. Peel the grapefruit, separate into segments, then add them to the vegetables. Pour the dressing over the salad and toss gently to combine.
4. Serve immediately or chill before serving. Enjoy!

Nutrition:

Per serving (based on 4 servings): Calories: 119; Total Fat: 8 g; Saturated Fat: 1 g; Cholesterol: 0 mg; Sodium: 53 mg; Carbohydrates: 10 g; Fiber: 3 g ; Sugar 7g ; Protein 2g.

QUICK HUMMUS AND GREEK SALAD

Cook Time: 15 minutes

Serving: 4-6 people

Ingredients:

- 1 can (15.5 oz) garbanzo beans, drained and rinsed
- 2 cloves garlic, minced
- 2 tablespoons tahini paste
- Juice of one lemon (2-3 tablespoons)
- 1/4 teaspoon ground cumin
- 1 tablespoon olive oil
- Salt and pepper to taste
- Cucumber, diced small
- Tomato, diced small
- Feta cheese, crumbled
- 2 tablespoons chopped fresh dill
- 2 tablespoons freshly squeezed orange juice

Preparation:

1. In a food processor or blender, combine the garbanzo beans, garlic, tahini paste, lemon juice, cumin and olive oil. Blend until creamy. If needed add 2-3 tablespoons of water to achieve desired consistency. Season with salt and pepper to taste.

2. Serve the hummus in a bowl and top with cucumber, tomato, feta cheese and dill. Drizzle orange juice over the top for an extra burst of flavor.
3. Enjoy your delicious Quick Hummus and Greek Salad!

Nutrition:

A serving size of quick hummus and Greek salad contains approximately 150 calories, 5g fat (1g saturated), 20g carbohydrates (6g fiber), 6g protein, 70mg sodium.

Enjoy your healthy and delicious snack!

QUICK PESTO CHICKEN SALAD WITH GREENS

Cook Time: 10 minutes

Servings: 4

Ingredients:

- 2 chicken breasts, cooked and shredded
- 1/4 cup pesto sauce
- 3 cups mixed green lettuce
- 1/2 cup cherry tomatoes, cut in half
- 1/2 red onion, thinly sliced
- Salt & pepper to taste

Preparation:

1. In a medium-sized bowl combine the shredded chicken, pesto sauce and salt & pepper. Mix until everything is evenly combined. Set aside.
2. Place the mixed greens in a large salad bowl or platter and top with the prepared chicken mixture. Sprinkle over onion slices and tomatoes and gently toss the salad.
3. Serve with additional dressing, if desired. Enjoy!

Nutrition:

Calories 218, Fat 13g, Carbohydrate 4g, Protein 18g.

CRISPY TOFU WITH VEGETABLE SALAD

Cook Time: 20 minutes

Serving: 4 people

Ingredients:

- 10 ounces extra-firm tofu, diced
- 2 tablespoons vegetable oil
- 1/3 cup all-purpose flour
- Salt and pepper to taste
- 2 tablespoons sesame oil
- 1/2 teaspoon garlic powder

For the Salad:

- 3 cups mixed greens of your choice
- 1 tablespoon olive oil
- 2 tablespoons balsamic vinegar or other vinaigrette of your choice

Preparation:

1. Preheat oven to 350°F (176°C). Place diced tofu in a large bowl. Drizzle on the vegetable oil and toss to evenly coat.
2. In a shallow dish, mix together the flour and salt and pepper. Dredge each piece of tofu in the flour mixture until completely coated.
3. Place on a parchment-lined baking sheet, drizzle with sesame oil, and sprinkle with garlic powder. Bake for 15

minutes or until golden brown, flipping halfway through cooking time.
4. While the tofu is baking, prepare your salad by combining all ingredients in a large bowl and tossing to combine. Serve the crispy tofu over the salad and enjoy!

Nutrition:

Serving size 1/4 of recipe | Calories: 159 kcal | Carbohydrates: 7g | Protein: 8g | Fat: 11g | Saturated Fat: 6g | Sodium: 19mg | Potassium: 48mg | Fiber: 1.3g | Sugar: 0.7g | Vitamin A: 16% | Vitamin C 6%. Iron 5%. Calcium 4%.

HEALTHY SPINACH SALAD

Cook Time: 10 minutes

Servings: 6-8 people

Ingredients:

- 4 cups baby spinach leaves
- 2 medium tomatoes, diced
- 1/2 cup cucumber slices
- 1 avocado, peeled and diced
- 1/4 cup slivered almonds
- 3 tablespoons olive oil
- 3 tablespoons white wine vinegar
- Salt to taste

Preparation:

- In a large salad bowl, combine the spinach, tomatoes, cucumbers and avocados together.
- Sprinkle the almonds over the top of the salad.
- Drizzle with olive oil and vinegar, then season with salt.
- Serve immediately or chill until ready to serve.

Nutrition:

This salad is a great source of vitamin A, vitamin C and fiber, as well as healthy fats from the avocado and olive oil. Enjoy!

ROASTED CHICKEN AND MUSHROOMS SALAD

Cook time: 20 minutes

Serving: 4

Ingredients:

- 2 tablespoons olive oil
- 1 pound chicken breast, cut into cubes
- 8 ounces mushrooms, sliced
- 1 teaspoon garlic powder
- 2 teaspoons Italian seasoning
- Salt and pepper to taste

Preparation:

1. Heat the olive oil in a large skillet over medium heat. Add the cubed chicken and cook until lightly browned on all sides. Cook for about 5 minutes.
2. Add the mushrooms to the skillet and season with garlic powder, Italian seasoning, salt and pepper. Stir to combine and continue cooking for an additional 7 to 10 minutes or until chicken is cooked through and mushrooms are golden brown.
3. Remove from heat and let cool before transferring to a bowl or platter to serve.

Nutrition:

Calories: 222, Fat: 10g, Protein: 26g, Carbs: 5g, Fiber: 2g, Sugar: 1g, Cholesterol: 72mg, Sodium: 106mg.

CHICKPEA, BROCCOLI, AND POMEGRANATE SALAD

Cook Time: 10 minutes

Servings: 4-6 servings

Ingredients:

- 2 cups cooked chickpeas, rinsed and drained
- 1 small head of broccoli, cut into small florets
- ½ cup pomegranate seeds
- ¼ cup diced red onion
- ¼ cup crumbled feta cheese (optional)
- 2 tablespoons extra virgin olive oil
- Juice from ½ a lemon
- Salt and pepper to taste

Preparation:

1. Preheat oven to 375°F (190°C). Spread chickpeas on one side of a baking sheet. On the other side spread out broccoli. Drizzle with olive oil and season with salt and pepper.
2. Bake for 10 minutes, stirring halfway through until broccoli is lightly golden brown and tender.
3. In a large bowl combine cooked chickpeas, roasted broccoli, pomegranate seeds, diced red onion, feta cheese (optional). Drizzle with lemon juice and remaining olive oil (if desired) and mix to combine.
4. Season with additional salt or pepper if needed and serve!

Nutrition:

1 serving of this Chickpea, Broccoli & Pomegranate Salad contains approximately 112 calories, 5 g fat, 13 g carbohydrate, 4 g protein, 3 g fiber and 189 mg sodium. Additionally it is an excellent source of vitamin C, phosphorus and iron. It is a good source of folate, magnesium, zinc and vitamin K. Enjoy!

ANCHOVY, ORANGE, AND OUVE SALAD

Cook Time: 10 minutes

Servings: Makes 4 servings

Ingredients:

- 1/2 cup chopped anchovies
- 2 oranges, segmented and sliced into thin rounds
- 1/4 cup pitted olives, coarsely chopped
- 2 tablespoons lemon juice
- 2 tablespoons olive oil
- Salt and freshly ground black pepper to taste

Preparation:

1. In a medium bowl, combine the anchovies, oranges, olives, lemon juice, and olive oil. Stir gently until all ingredients are combined.
2. Season with salt and pepper to taste. Serve chilled or at room temperature. Enjoy!

Nutrition:

Per Serving - Calories (171), Total Fat (11 g), Saturated Fat (2 g), Cholesterol (12 mg), Sodium (465 mg), Carbohydrates (14 g) Protein (3 g).

VEGETABLE AND CHICKPEA SALAD

Cook Time: 20 minutes

Servings: 4-6

Ingredients:

- 2 cups diced cooked vegetables (such as carrots, potatoes, beans)
- 1 cup cooked chickpeas
- 2 tablespoons olive oil
- Salt and pepper to taste
- 1 tablespoon chopped fresh herbs such as thyme or oregano (optional)

Preparation:

1. In a medium bowl, combine the cooked vegetables and chickpeas. Drizzle with olive oil, salt and pepper. Mix to combine until all ingredients are well coated.
2. Place in a serving dish and garnish with fresh herbs, if desired. Serve warm or cold. Enjoy!

Nutrition:

This salad is a great source of protein, healthy fats and complex carbohydrates. It is also low in calories and fat, making it a great healthy side dish. It contains vitamins A, C and B6 as well as minerals such as iron, magnesium and potassium. Enjoy!

TABOULI WITH VEGGIES SALAD

Cook time: 15 minutes

Serving: 4 people

Ingredients:

- 2 cups of bulgur wheat
- 1 medium onion, finely diced
- 2 tomatoes, seeded and diced
- 1 cucumber, seeded and diced
- 1/4 cup fresh chopped parsley
- 2 tablespoons extra virgin olive oil
- Juice from 1 lemon (about 3 tablespoons)
- Salt and pepper to taste

Preparation:

1. Rinse the bulgur wheat in cold water until it is completely clean. Drain, then add to a large bowl with 2 cups of hot boiling water. Let sit for 10 minutes or until softened. Drain off any excess liquid.
2. In a separate bowl, mix together the diced onion, tomatoes, cucumber and parsley.
3. Add the softened bulgur wheat to the vegetables, along with the olive oil, lemon juice and salt and pepper. Mix well to combine all of the ingredients.
4. Serve immediately or refrigerate for up to 4 days in an airtight container.

Nutrition:

This tabouli salad is a good source of protein, fiber, minerals and vitamins A and C. It's also low in calories and fat so it makes a great side dish or light lunch option! Enjoy!

HEALTHY FATTOUSH SALAD

Cook Time: 15 minutes

Servings: 6-8

Ingredients:

- 2 medium heads of romaine lettuce, chopped into bite-sized pieces
- 2 large tomatoes, diced
- 1/2 cucumber, peeled and diced
- 1/4 red onion, thinly sliced
- 4 green onions (scallions), finely chopped
- 1/4 cup fresh parsley leaves, finely chopped
- 1/4 cup fresh mint leaves, finely chopped
- 3 tablespoons olive oil
- Juice from 1 lemon

Preparation:

1. In a large bowl combine the lettuce, tomatoes, cucumber, red onion and green onions. In a smaller bowl whisk together the parsley, mint, olive oil and lemon juice. Pour the dressing over the salad ingredients and toss to combine.

Nutrition:

This healthy fattoush salad is a great way to get your daily servings of vegetables! Each serving provides 100 calories, 7g fat, 5g carbs, and 2g protein. It's also high in vitamins A & C as well as dietary fiber. Enjoy!

VEGGIES WITH CHICKPEA SALAD

Cook Time: 10 minutes

Serving: 4-6 people

Ingredients:

- 2 cans chickpeas, drained and rinsed
- 3 cups fresh veggies of your choice (e.g. carrot, cucumber, bell pepper) finely chopped
- ¼ cup olive oil
- 2 tablespoons fresh lemon juice
- 3 cloves garlic, minced
- 2 tablespoons fresh basil, finely chopped
- 1 teaspoon sea salt
- ½ teaspoon black pepper

Preparation:

2. In a large mixing bowl, combine the chickpeas and chopped vegetables.
3. In a separate small bowl, whisk together olive oil, lemon juice, garlic, basil, salt and pepper until combined. Pour this dressing over the chickpea and vegetable mixture and toss to combine.
4. Serve chilled or at room temperature as is or with your favorite accompaniment such as crackers or pita bread! Enjoy!

Nutrition:

This delicious salad provides lots of fiber from the chickpeas and an array of vitamins, minerals and antioxidants from the fresh vegetables.

CHEESY SCRAMBLED EGGS WITH FRESH HERBS

Cook Time: 10 minutes

Servings: 4

Ingredients:

- 2 tablespoons butter or olive oil
- 6 large eggs
- 1/4 cup milk
- 1/4 teaspoon garlic powder
- 1/4 teaspoon onion powder
- Salt and pepper, to taste
- 2 tablespoons freshly chopped herbs (parsley, chives, thyme)

Preparation:

1. Heat a medium skillet over medium heat and add the butter or olive oil. Once melted, add in the eggs and scramble until just set.
2. Add in the milk, garlic powder, onion powder, salt and pepper. Continue to scramble until all ingredients are combined and eggs are cooked through.
3. Remove eggs from the heat and stir in fresh herbs. Serve immediately with your favorite toast or side dish.

Nutrition:

Calories: 122 kcal, Carbohydrates: 1 g, Protein: 8 g, Fat: 9 g, Saturated Fat: 4 g, Cholesterol: 213 mg, Sodium: 97 mg,

Potassium: 105 mg, Sugar: 1 g, Vitamin A: 590 IU, Calcium: 59 mg Iron : 1 mg.

POULTRY AND MEAT

CHICKEN AND LEMONGRASS SAUCE

Cook Time: 15 minutes

Servings: 4

Ingredients:

- 2 tablespoons olive oil
- 2 cloves garlic, minced
- 1/2 teaspoon ground ginger
- 2 boneless skinless chicken breasts, cut into cubes
- 1/4 cup low-sodium soy sauce
- 1 tablespoon fish sauce
- 1 lime, juiced
- 1 stalk lemongrass, thinly sliced and crushed

Preparation:

1. Heat the olive oil in a large skillet over medium heat. Add the garlic and ginger and cook for about 30 seconds until fragrant.
2. Add the chicken and cook for 5 minutes until golden brown. Stir in the soy sauce, fish sauce, and lime juice.
3. Add the lemongrass and cook for another 5 minutes until the chicken is cooked through.
4. Serve over hot white rice or noodles.

Nutrition:

Per Serving: Calories 155; Fat 6g; Carbohydrates 4g; Protein 19g; Cholesterol 45mg; Sodium 824mg; Fiber 1g; Sugar 2g.

SESAME CHICKEN WITH BLACK RICE, BROCCOLI, AND SNAP PEAS

Cook Time: 30 minutes

Servings: 4

Ingredients:

- 2 tablespoons olive oil
- 1/2 cup diced onion
- 1 pound boneless skinless chicken breast, cut into bite size pieces
- 3 cloves garlic, minced
- 2 tablespoons soy sauce or tamari gluten free soy sauce if needed
- 1 tablespoon honey
- 1 teaspoon sesame oil
- 1/4 teaspoon ground ginger
- Salt and pepper to taste
- 3 cups cooked black rice (or your favorite kind of rice)
- 2 cups broccoli florets
- 2 cups snap peas (snow peas are a good substitute)

Preparation:

- Heat the olive oil in a large skillet over medium-high heat.
- Add the onion, chicken and garlic to the pan, season with salt and pepper and cook for about 8 minutes or until the chicken is cooked through.
- Stir in the soy sauce or tamari, honey, sesame oil and ground ginger. Cook for 1 minute more.
- In a separate pot, cook rice according to package instructions then add it to your skillet with the vegetables.

- Add the broccoli and snap peas to the skillet and cook for an additional 5 minutes or until all of the ingredients are heated through and cooked to your desired texture level.
- Serve warm with steamed white rice or brown rice.

Nutrition:

One serving of this Sesame Chicken with Black Rice, Broccoli and Snap Peas recipe contains about 349 calories, 4g fat, 45g protein, 42g carbs, and 8g fiber. It also provides you with a good source of vitamins A & C as well as iron and calcium. Enjoy!

TASTY LAMB RIBS

Cook time: 1 hour 30 minutes

Serving size: 4-6 people

Ingredients:

- 2-3 lbs of lamb ribs
- 2 teaspoons of garlic powder
- 1 teaspoon of onion powder
- 2 tablespoons of olive oil
- 2 tablespoons of salt
- 3 tablespoons of fresh cracked pepper
- ½ cup of honey BBQ sauce (or your favorite BBQ sauce)

Preparation:

1. Preheat your oven to 375° F. Grease a large baking sheet with olive oil.
2. Lay out the ribs on the prepared baking sheet, season them with garlic and onion powder, salt, and pepper. Make sure the ribs are evenly coated all around with the spices.
3. Drizzle olive oil over the top of the ribs, then rub it over them to create a thin layer.
4. Bake in preheated oven for 1 hour 30 minutes, flipping once halfway through cooking time.
5. Once they're done baking, brush BBQ sauce all over them and bake an additional 5-10 minutes until bubbly and golden brown on top.

6. Slice into individual portions and serve hot!

Nutrition Information:

Calories: 456 kcal Carbohydrates: 22g Protein: 35g Fat: 24g Saturated Fat: 8g Cholesterol: 96mg Sodium: 1375mg Potassium: 582mg Fiber: 1g Sugar: 16g Vitamin A: 68IU Calcium: 55mg Iron: 2.2mg Enjoy your delicious lamb ribs! They make for a great meal and are sure to please the entire family. Serve with some mashed potatoes and vegetables for a complete dinner.

SAFFRON BEEF

Cook Time: 30 minutes

Serving Size: 2-3 people

Ingredients:
- 1 pound beef sirloin, cut into thin strips
- 3 tablespoons vegetable oil
- 2 shallots, peeled and diced
- 2 cloves garlic, minced
- 1 teaspoon freshly grated ginger root
- 2 teaspoons paprika
- 1 teaspoon turmeric powder
- ½ teaspoon ground cinnamon
- Pinch of cayenne pepper (optional)
- Salt and pepper to taste

Preparation:
1. Season the beef with salt and pepper. Heat the oil in a large skillet over medium heat. Add the beef slices and cook for 5 to 6 minutes, stirring frequently.
2. Add the shallots and garlic to the skillet. Cook for another 3 to 4 minutes or until vegetables are softened.
3. Stir in the ginger, paprika, turmeric powder, cinnamon and cayenne pepper (if using). Cook for an additional minute or two until fragrant.

4. Reduce heat to low and simmer for 15-20 minutes, stirring occasionally, until beef is cooked through and sauce has thickened slightly.
5. Serve with steamed white rice or noodles and your favorite sides such as carrots or broccoli florets. Enjoy!

Nutrition:

Per serving (based on 3 servings): Calories: 374; Total Fat: 14.7g; Saturated Fat: 5.4g; Cholesterol: 83mg; Sodium: 263mg; Carbohydrate: 8.9g; Dietary Fiber: 1.3g; Protein: 45.2g.

CHICKEN AND BUTTER SAUCE

Cook Time: 10 minutes

Servings: 4

Ingredients:

- 1 tablespoon butter
- 2 cloves garlic, minced
- 1/2 teaspoon dried oregano
- 1/2 teaspoon dried basil
- Salt and pepper to taste
- 1 pound boneless skinless chicken breasts, cut into bite size pieces
- 2 tablespoons all purpose flour
- 2 tablespoons white wine or chicken broth.

Preparation:

1. Heat the butter in a large skillet over medium heat. Once melted, add the garlic and sauté until fragrant, about 30 seconds.
2. Add the oregano, basil, salt, and pepper, then stir to combine.
3. Add the chicken pieces and cook until lightly browned on all sides, about 7-10 minutes.
4. Sprinkle the flour over the chicken and stir to coat evenly; cook for 1 minute more.

5. Pour in the wine or broth and bring to a boil; reduce heat and simmer for 3-5 minutes until sauce has thickened.
6. Serve with your favorite side dishes and enjoy!

Nutrition Information:

One serving of this recipe contains approximately 217 calories, 9 grams of fat, 20 grams of protein, 8 grams carbohydrate, and 2 grams fiber.

LEMON AND GARLIC BARBECUED OCEAN TROUT WITH GREEN SALAD

Cook Time: 20 minutes

Serving: Makes 4 servings

Ingredients:

- 1 whole ocean trout, approximately 2 pounds
- 3 tablespoons olive oil
- 1 lemon, thinly sliced
- 2 cloves garlic, minced
- 1/2 teaspoon salt
- 1/4 teaspoon black pepper
- 8 cups mixed greens or salad of choice (cherry tomatoes, cucumbers, etc.)

Preparation:

1. Preheat your oven to 350°F. Line a baking sheet with parchment paper and place the fish on it.
2. Rub the olive oil over the fish and set aside the remaining oil for later. Place the lemon slices on top of the fish and sprinkle the minced garlic over it. Season with salt and pepper.
3. Bake in preheated oven for 15 minutes or until the fish is cooked through.

4. Meanwhile, prepare your salad by tossing together mixed greens or whatever combination of vegetables you prefer with the remaining olive oil, salt and pepper to taste.
5. Plate the Trout on top of a bed of green salad and serve immediately!

Nutrition:

Per Serving : Calories 249, Total Fats 11g, Saturated Fat 2g, Cholesterol 56mg, Sodium 488mg, Carbohydrates 5g, Dietary Fiber 2g, Sugars 1g, Protein 28g.

CHICKEN AND BLACK BEANS

Cook time: 15 minutes

Serving: 4 people

Ingredients:
- 1 can (14.5 oz) black beans, drained and rinsed
- 1 cup chicken broth
- 1/2 red bell pepper, diced
- 2 cloves garlic, minced
- 1 teaspoon chili powder
- Salt and pepper to taste

Preparation:
1. Heat a large skillet over medium heat. Add the bell pepper and garlic and cook for about 5 minutes or until softened.
2. Add the chili powder and stir to combine. Then add the chicken broth, black beans, and salt and pepper to taste. Simmer for 10 minutes uncovered or until most of the liquid is absorbed.
3. Serve over cooked rice or quinoa and garnish with fresh cilantro, if desired.

Nutrition:
Serving size 1/4 of recipe | Calories 195 | Total fat 2g | Saturated fat 0g | Cholesterol 9mg | Sodium 578mg | Total carbohydrate 31g | Dietary fiber 10g| Sugars 4g| Protein 13g

SWEET CHIPOTLE GRILLED BEEF RIBS

Cook Time: Approximately 1 hour and 15 minutes

Servings: 4

Ingredients:

- 2 pounds beef ribs (back or short)
- ¼ cup Sweet Chipotle Spice Rub
- ½ cup of your favorite BBQ sauce

Preparation:

1. Preheat the oven to 350°F. Line a baking sheet with aluminum foil.

2. Pat the ribs dry with paper towels, then rub them all over with the Sweet Chipotle Spice Rub, making sure it gets into any crevices in the meat. Place on the prepared baking sheet, cover with aluminum foil and bake for 45 minutes. Remove from oven and let cool slightly before handling.

3. Preheat an outdoor grill to medium-high heat. Place ribs onto the hot grate, close the lid and cook for 10–15 minutes, flipping once or twice.

4. Brush the ribs with your favorite BBQ sauce and continue to cook over medium-high heat until they reach an internal temperature of 160°F when tested with a meat thermometer.

5. Serve warm!

Nutrition:

Each serving contains approximately 500 calories, 16g fat, 38g carbohydrates and 32g protein.

GRILLED SIRLOIN STEAK WITH SAUCE DIANE

Cook Time: 25 minutes

Serving: 4 people

Ingredients:

- 4 (7-8 ounce) boneless sirloin steaks, 1 inch thick
- 2 tablespoons butter
- 2 tablespoons shallots, minced
- 1 cup beef stock or broth
- 1/4 cup brandy or cognac
- 2 tablespoons Dijon mustard
- 2 teaspoons Worcestershire sauce
- Salt and pepper to taste

Preparation:

1. Heat a heavy skillet over medium heat. Add the butter and shallots and sauté until the shallot is softened. Remove the pan from the heat.
2. Rub both sides of the steaks with salt and pepper. Place the steak in the skillet and cook for about 5 minutes on each side, or until done to your liking.
3. Remove the steak from the pan and keep warm.
4. Add the beef stock or broth to the skillet and bring to a boil over high heat. Simmer for 23 minutes, stirring occasionally.

5. Reduce the heat to low and add the brandy, mustard, Worcestershire sauce, salt, and pepper; stir to combine all ingredients together. Let simmer for a few minutes until slightly thickened and reduced by half in volume.
6. Return steaks to pan along with any accumulated juices; spoon sauce over the steaks.
7. Simmer for 1-2 minutes to heat through and coat with sauce.
8. Serve steaks with sauce drizzled over top.

Nutrition:

Calories: 343 kcal, Carbohydrates: 1 g, Protein: 35 g, Fat 17 g, Saturated Fat 8 g, Cholesterol 116 mg Sodium 327 mg Potassium 635 mg Fiber 0g Sugar 0g Vitamin A 134 IU Vitamin C 1.3 mg Calcium 24 mg Iron 3.5mg.

RIB ROAST WITH ROASTED SHALLOTS AND GARLIC

Cook Time: 40 minutes

Servings: 4-6

Ingredients:

- 2 to 3lb rib roast
- 5 shallots, peeled and quartered
- 4 cloves of garlic, peeled and minced
- 2 tablespoons extra virgin olive oil
- Salt and pepper to taste

Preparation:

1. Preheat oven to 350°F. Rub the roast with some of the olive oil and season liberally with salt and pepper. Place in a roasting pan or baking dish. Peel and quarter the shallots; mince the garlic cloves. Scatter them around the meat in the pan. Drizzle remaining olive oil over vegetables. Cover with foil or a lid and place in preheated oven.

2. Roast for 25 minutes, basting occasionally with pan juices, then remove lid or foil and roast uncovered for an additional 15 minutes until internal temperature registers 145°F on a meat thermometer. Let rest at least 10 minutes before carving. Serve with roasted shallots and garlic.

Nutrition Facts:

Per Serving (based on 4 servings): Calories 425, Fat 29g (Saturated 10g), Cholesterol 135mg, Sodium 117mg, Carbohydrate 3g, Fiber 1g, Sugar 0g, Protein 36g. Enjoy!

BEEF MEATBALLS

Cook Time: 15 minutes

Serving Size: 4-6 people

Ingredients:

- 1 lb. Ground beef
- ½ cup Panko breadcrumbs
- 1 teaspoon garlic powder
- 2 eggs, beaten
- ¼ cup chopped fresh parsley
- Salt and pepper to taste

Preparation:

- Preheat the oven to 375 degrees Fahrenheit. Line a baking sheet with parchment paper or grease lightly with cooking spray.
- In a large bowl, combine ground beef, panko breadcrumbs, garlic powder, eggs and parsley until just combined. Season generously with salt and pepper.
- Form beef mixture into 1-inch meatballs and place on prepared baking sheet.
- Bake in preheated oven for 15 minutes or until the internal temperature of the meatballs reaches 165 degrees Fahrenheit. Serve warm with your favorite sauce and sides!

Nutrition

(per serving): Calories: 250; Fat: 12g; Saturated Fat: 5g; Protein: 25g; Carbohydrates: 9g; Fiber: 1g; Sodium: 170mg. Enjoy!

POT ROAST

Cook Time: 3-4 hours

Serving Size: 4-6 people

Ingredients:

- 2-3 pound beef chuck roast
- 1 onion, sliced
- 3 cloves of garlic, minced
- 2 tablespoons olive oil
- Salt and pepper to taste
- 2 cups beef broth or stock
- 1 tablespoon Worcestershire sauce

Preparation:

1. Preheat oven to 300°F (150°C). Heat the olive oil in a large skillet over medium heat. Add the onion and garlic and cook until golden brown. Set aside.
2. Season the beef with salt and pepper. Place the beef in the skillet and sear on all sides.
3. Transfer the beef to a roasting pan. Add the onion, garlic, and beef broth. Cover with foil and place in preheated oven for 3-4 hours or until tender.
4. Remove from oven and let rest for 10 minutes before slicing against the grain.

Nutrition:

Calories: 500 kcal | Carbohydrates: 5 g | Protein: 35 g | Fat: 36 g | Saturated Fat: 12 g | Cholesterol: 142 mg | Sodium: 441 mg | Potassium: 755 mg | Fiber: 1 g| Sugar: 1g | Vitamin A: 28 IU | Vitamin C: 2 mg | Calcium: 63 mg | Iron: 6 mg .Enjoy!

BEEF TRIPE POT

Cook Time: 1 hour 40 minutes

Servings: 4

Ingredients:

- 2 lbs beef tripe, cut into small cubes
- 3 cloves garlic, minced
- 1 onion, diced
- 1 red bell pepper, sliced
- 3 tablespoons olive oil
- ¼ cup white wine vinegar
- 2 cups beef stock
- 1 teaspoon paprika
- 2 tablespoons tomato paste
- Salt and black pepper to taste

Preparation:

1. Heat the olive oil in a large pot over medium heat. Add the garlic and onions and cook until softened, about 5 minutes. Add the bell pepper and cook for another 3 minutes.

2. Add the beef tripe and cook until browned, about 5 minutes. Pour in the white wine vinegar and cook for an additional 2 minutes.

3. Stir in the beef stock, paprika, tomato paste, and season with salt and pepper to taste.

4. Bring to a boil then reduce heat to low and simmer for 1 hour 30 minutes.
5. Serve hot over cooked rice or mashed potatoes. Enjoy!

Nutrition:

Per Serving (1/4 of recipe): Calories: 314; Fat: 18g; Carbohydrates: 6g; Protein: 24g; Cholesterol: 69mg; Sodium: 191mg; Fiber: 1g.

LOVELY PULLED CHICKEN EGG BITES

Cook Time: 10 minutes

Servings: 4

Ingredients:

- 2 tablespoons olive oil
- 1 medium onion, chopped
- 1 large garlic clove, minced
- ½ teaspoon ground cumin
- ¼ teaspoon chili powder
- 2 cups pulled cooked chicken (or use canned)
- 8 eggs, lightly beaten

Preparation:

1. Heat the olive oil in a large skillet over medium heat. Add the onion and sauté until softened, about 3 minutes. Add the garlic, cumin, and chili powder; stir until fragrant, about 30 seconds.
2. Stir in the chicken and cook for another minute or two to heat through.
3. Pour in the eggs, stirring lightly with a fork to break up any big chunks of chicken and scramble everything together. Cook for about 3 minutes until the eggs are set, stirring occasionally.
4. Serve hot or cold with your favorite sides. Enjoy!

Nutrition:

Calories: 227 kcal | Carbohydrates: 4 g | Protein: 18 g | Fat: 15 g | Saturated Fat: 3 g | Cholesterol: 222 mg | Sodium: 158 mg | Potassium: 246 mg | Fiber: 1g | Sugar: 2g| Vitamin A: 291 IU| Vitamin C 3mg| Calcium 52mg| Iron 2mg.

FISH AND SEAFOOD

SHRIMP WITH GARUC

Cook time: 10 minutes

Serving: 4 people

Ingredients:

- 500 g shrimps, deveined and shelled
- 1 tablespoon garuc paste
- 2 tablespoons olive oil
- 2 cloves garlic, finely chopped
- Salt and pepper to taste

Preparation:

1. Heat the olive oil in a pan over medium heat. Add the garlic and cook for 1 minute.
2. Add the garuc paste and cook for another minute.
3. Add the shrimps to the pan and season with salt and pepper. Cook until the shrimps turn pink, about 3 - 5 minutes.
4. Serve the shrimps with the garuc sauce.

Nutrition Info:

Serving size of 1 cup (160g): Calories: 123, Total Fat: 5g, Saturated Fat: 0.5g, Cholesterol: 193mg, Sodium: 187mg, Total Carbohydrate: 2g, Protein: 17.3g.

SABICH SANDWICH

Cook Time: 25 minutes

Servings: 2-4

Ingredients:

- 3 eggs
- 2 large potatoes, boiled and cubed
- 1/2 red onion, chopped
- 4 tablespoons of oil for frying (olive or vegetable)
- 1 tablespoon of mayonnaise, plus more to serve (optional)
- 2 small pita pockets or flatbreads, split in half and lightly grilled or toasted
- 1 cucumber, sliced into thin rounds
- 1 tomato, diced small
- Pickles or olives (optional)

Preparation:

1. Heat the oil in a pan over medium heat. Once hot, add the eggs and fry until cooked through, about 4 minutes.
2. Add the potatoes and onion to the pan and cook for an additional 2-3 minutes, stirring often.
3. Once everything is cooked through, turn off the heat. Assemble each pita pocket by adding a few spoonful's of egg and potato mixture, mayonnaise (optional), cucumber slices, tomato, pickles or olives if desired.
4. Serve warm with extra mayonnaise on the side (optional).

Nutrition:

This SABICH sandwich contains approximately 380 calories per serving and is high in protein and iron due to the addition of eggs. It is a good source of vitamins A, C & K from the added vegetables. The mayonnaise adds an additional 100 calories and 10 grams of fat to each serving. Enjoy!

SALMON WITH VEGETABLES

Cook Time: 15 minutes

Servings: 4

Ingredients:
- 4 (6 oz) salmon fillets
- 1 tbsp garlic powder
- 1 tsp onion powder
- Salt and pepper to taste
- 2 tbsp olive oil
- 2 cups diced vegetables of your choice (such as bell peppers, zucchini, carrots, mushrooms, etc.)

Preparation:
1. Preheat oven to 375°F. Grease a baking dish large enough for all four pieces of salmon and set aside.
2. In a small bowl combine the garlic powder, onion powder, salt and pepper; mix together and set aside.
3. Rub each piece of salmon with olive oil and sprinkle the seasoning mixture over each piece. Place salmon fillets in a single layer in the baking dish.
4. Bake for 10 minutes, then add vegetables of your choice around the salmon. Sprinkle with additional seasonings if desired.
5. Cook for an additional 5 minutes until the fish is cooked through and the vegetables are tender-crisp.

Nutrition:

Salmon is a great source of protein, healthy fats, vitamins and minerals such as omega-3 fatty acids, B12 and selenium. When paired with nutritious vegetables this meal provides a balanced combination of nutrient dense ingredients that will support overall health and wellness! Enjoy!

CRISPY FISH

Cook Time: 15 minutes

Serving Size: 4-6 servings

Ingredients

- 1.5 pounds of a white flaky fish (cod, haddock, or tilapia)
- 2 teaspoons Cajun seasoning blend
- 1/4 teaspoon garlic powder
- 2 tablespoons all-purpose flour
- 2 tablespoons olive oil

Preparation:

1. Preheat oven to 425 F (220C). Line a baking sheet with parchment paper and set aside.
2. Cut the fish into four equal pieces, making sure to remove any small bones that may be present. Place the fish on the prepared baking sheet.
3. In a small bowl, combine the Cajun seasoning blend and garlic powder. Sprinkle the mixture evenly over both sides of each piece of fish.
4. Place flour in a shallow dish or plate and coat each side of the fish with it.
5. Heat olive oil in a large skillet over medium-high heat until hot and place the fish into the pan for about 2 minutes per side, until golden brown and crisp on both sides.

6. Transfer to prepared baking sheet and bake for 10-12 minutes, until cooked through and flaky inside. Serve warm with lemon wedges if desired!

Nutrition:

Calories: 224; Total Fat: 9g; Saturated Fat: 1g; Cholesterol: 69mg; Sodium: 327mg; Total Carbohydrates: 3g; Dietary Fiber: 0.5g; Protein: 30.6g.

MOULES MARINIERES

Cook Time: 10 minutes

Servings: 4

Ingredients:

- 2 pounds of cleaned mussels
- 1 tablespoon of olive oil
- 2 shallots, finely chopped
- 2 cloves of garlic, minced
- 1/2 cup dry white wine
- 3 tablespoons unsalted butter
- 2 teaspoons fresh thyme leaves
- Salt and pepper to taste

Preparation:

1. Heat the olive oil in a large pot over medium heat. Add the shallots and garlic and cook until softened, about 3 minutes.
2. Increase the heat to high and add in the mussels. Stir for 2 minutes, then pour in the white wine and butter.
3. Cover with a lid and steam for 5 minutes until all of the mussels have opened up. Discard any that did not open.
4. Sprinkle with thyme leaves, season with salt and pepper to taste, then serve immediately.

Nutrition:

One serving of Moules marinières contains approximately 340 calories, 17 grams of fat, 21 grams of carbohydrates, 16 grams of protein and 1.5 grams of dietary fiber. It is also a good source of iron and vitamin B12.

STEAMED MUSSELS WITH COCONUT-CURRY

Cook time: 10 minutes

Serving: 4 people

Ingredients:

- 2 lbs mussels, cleaned and debearded
- 2 tablespoons coconut oil or olive oil
- 1/2 teaspoon curry powder
- 1 cup of canned coconut milk
- Juice from one lime or lemon (optional)
- Salt and freshly ground pepper to taste

Preparation:

1. Heat the oil in a large pot over medium heat. Add the curry powder and stir for about 30 seconds until fragrant.
2. Pour in the coconut milk and bring it to a boil, then reduce the heat to low and simmer for 5 minutes.
3. Add the mussels to the pot and cover with a lid. Cook for 5 minutes until all of the mussels have opened.
4. Add the lime or lemon juice, salt, and pepper if needed, then serve hot!

Nutrition Information

(per serving): Calories: 144 kcal Total Fat: 11 g Saturated Fat: 8 g Cholesterol: 53 mg Sodium: 495 mg Carbohydrates: 4 g Protein: 10 g Fiber: 0g With this recipe, you'll have delicious steamed mussels in no time at all! Enjoy!

TUNA NOODLE CASSEROLE

Cook time: 30 minutes

Servings: 4-6 people

Ingredients:

- 2 tablespoons butter
- 1 onion, diced
- 1 (10.75 ounce) can cream of mushroom soup
- 1 (10.75 ounce) can cream of chicken soup
- 1 cup mayonnaise or Miracle Whip dressing
- 2 (3.5 ounce) cans tuna, drained and flaked
- 4 ounces uncooked egg noodles
- ¼ teaspoon ground black pepper
- ½ cup shredded Cheddar cheese, divided

Preparation:

1. Preheat oven to 350 degrees F (175 degrees C). Grease a 9x13 inch baking dish. Melt butter in a skillet over medium heat. Stir in onion, and cook until tender, about 5 minutes.

2. In a large bowl, mix together the mushroom soup, chicken soup, mayonnaise or Miracle Whip dressing, tuna, egg noodles, pepper and ¼ cup of cheese; stir in the cooked onions. Pour into baking dish. Sprinkle remaining cheese on top.

3. Bake uncovered for 25 to 30 minutes at 350 degrees F (175 degrees C) until bubbly and lightly browned on top.

Nutrition Information:

Per serving: Calories 394; Fat 21g; Protein 18g; Carbohydrate 29g; Fiber 2g; Cholesterol 53mg; Sodium 846mg.

SAUMON BURGERS

Cook Time: 20 minutes

Servings: 4 Burgers

Ingredients:

- 1 pound of ground salmon
- 2 cloves garlic, minced
- ¼ cup onion, diced small
- ½ teaspoon chili powder
- 1 teaspoon smoked paprika
- Salt and pepper to taste
- 2 tablespoons olive oil

Preparation:

1. Preheat oven to 425°F (220°C). Grease a baking sheet with cooking spray or line it with parchment paper.
2. In a medium bowl, combine the ground salmon, garlic, onion, chili powder, smoked paprika, salt and pepper. Mix until all ingredients are evenly distributed.
3. Divide the salmon mixture into 4 equal portions, and shape each portion into a patty.
4. Heat the olive oil in a large skillet over medium-high heat. Cook the burger patties for 3-4 minutes on each side, or until cooked through.
5. Place the burgers onto the prepared baking sheet and bake for 5 minutes, or until heated through.
6. Serve with your favorite sides and enjoy!

Nutrition:

Each burger provides approximately 285 calories, 15g of fat, 24g of protein, 1g of carbohydrates and 0g dietary fiber. Enjoy!

SEARED SCALLOPS

Cook Time: 6 minutes

Serving: 2 people

Ingredients:

- 12 large scallops
- 1 tablespoon olive oil
- 1 teaspoon salt
- ½ teaspoon black pepper
- 2 cloves garlic, minced
- 2 tablespoons butter

Preparation:

1. Heat a large non-stick skillet over medium-high heat.
2. Add the olive oil and scallops to the pan and season with salt and pepper. Cook for 3 minutes per side, or until golden brown and cooked through.
3. Add the garlic and butter to the pan. Swirl until melted and combined.
4. Serve immediately while hot with your favorite sides. Enjoy!

Nutrition:

Each serving contains approximately 156 calories, 10g fat, 2g carbohydrates, 13g protein. This dish is also a great source of B vitamins, iron, zinc, selenium and magnesium. Happy cooking! Now that you know how to get started with commands, try this recipe out for yourself – we're sure you'll love it!

BLACK COD

Cook Time: Prep time 5 minutes, cook time 10 minutes

Serving: 2 servings

Ingredients:

- 1 tablespoon olive oil
- 2 tablespoons black pepper
- 4 cloves garlic, minced
- 1 teaspoon dried oregano
- 1/4 cup red wine vinegar
- 1/2 teaspoon sea salt

Preparation:

1. Heat the olive oil in a skillet on medium heat. Add the garlic and sauté for one minute until fragrant. Add the black pepper, oregano, and sea salt to the pan and sauté for another minute.
2. Stir in the red wine vinegar, reduce heat to low and simmer for 5 minutes until the mixture is thickened.
3. Remove from heat and serve over cooked pasta, fish or chicken.

Nutrition:

Per Serving (1/2 cup): Calories: 97; Total Fat: 7g; Saturated Fat: 1g; Cholesterol: 0mg; Sodium: 394mg; Carbohydrates: 5g; Fiber: 2g; Sugar: 0g; Protein: 2g. Enjoy!

MISO-GLAZED SALMON

Cook Time: Total cook time is 20 minutes.

Servings: Makes 4 servings.

Ingredients:

- 4 6-oz salmon fillets
- 2 tablespoons miso paste
- 2 tablespoons honey or maple syrup
- 1 teaspoon sesame oil
- ½ teaspoon freshly grated ginger

Preparation:

- Preheat the oven to 375°F (190°C).
- Line a baking sheet with parchment paper and place the salmon fillets on it.
- In a small bowl, mix together the miso paste, honey or maple syrup, sesame oil and grated ginger until smooth.
- Spread the miso mixture evenly over the salmon fillets.
- Bake in the preheated oven for 15-20 minutes, until the salmon is cooked through and flaky.
- Serve immediately with your favorite sides.

Nutrition Info:

Calories 259, Total Fat 8 g, Saturated Fat 2 g, Cholesterol 93 mg, Sodium 492 mg, Carbohydrates 11 g, Protein 33 g.

ARUGULA AND SWEET POTATO SALAD

Cook Time: 30 minutes

Serving Size: 4-6 people

Ingredients:

- 2 sweet potatoes, diced into small cubes
- 1/4 cup olive oil
- 3 tablespoons white balsamic vinegar
- 1 teaspoon salt
- 1/4 teaspoon freshly ground black pepper
- 2 cloves garlic, minced
- 3 cups fresh arugula leaves, washed and dried
- 1/2 cup feta cheese, crumbled (optional)

Preparation:

1. Preheat the oven to 400°F. Line a baking sheet with parchment paper or aluminum foil. Place the diced sweet potatoes onto the baking sheet in an even layer. Drizzle with 2 tablespoons of the olive oil and toss with a spatula to evenly coat. Roast for 20-25 minutes, flipping halfway through cooking, until lightly golden brown.

2. Meanwhile, in a large bowl whisk together the remaining 2 tablespoons of olive oil, white balsamic vinegar, salt, pepper and minced garlic to make the dressing.

3. Add the roasted sweet potatoes into the bowl with the dressing and toss to combine. Let sit for 5 minutes to let all the flavors meld together.
4. Just before serving add in the arugula leaves and feta cheese (if using). Toss once more to combine everything together and serve!

Nutrition:

Per Serving – Calories: 126, Fat: 8.8g, Carbohydrates: 11.6g, Fiber: 2.4g, Protein: 2.3g Enjoy!

SHRIMP CURRY

Cook time: 15 minutes

Serving: 4 servings

Ingredients:

- 1 lb peeled and deveined shrimp, tail-off
- 2 tablespoons olive oil or ghee
- 2 cloves garlic, minced
- 1 teaspoon ground coriander
- ½ teaspoon ground cumin
- ½ teaspoon smoked paprika
- ¼ teaspoon turmeric powder
- 1/8 teaspoon chili powder (optional)
- 2 teaspoons ginger paste or grated fresh ginger
- 1 cup diced tomatoes
- 1 tablespoon tomato paste
- ¼ cup coconut milk or heavy cream

Preparation:

1. Heat the oil in a large skillet over medium heat. Once hot, add the garlic and cook for 1 minute until fragrant.
2. Add the ground coriander, cumin, smoked paprika, turmeric powder and chili powder (if using) to the pan and mix with a wooden spoon. Cook for 2 minutes, stirring occasionally.

3. Add the peeled shrimp to the pan along with ginger paste or grated fresh ginger and cook for 3-4 minutes until lightly cooked but not too firm in texture.
4. Add diced tomatoes, tomato paste and coconut milk or heavy cream to the pan and stir everything together. Let simmer on low heat for 5-7 minutes or until sauce has thickened slightly and shrimp is fully cooked through. Taste and adjust seasoning if needed with salt and pepper.
5. Serve curry with steamed basmati rice or your favorite grain. Enjoy!

Nutrition

(per serving): Calories: 263, Fat: 10g, Carbs: 4g, Protein: 32g, Fiber: 1g, Sugar: 1.5g, Sodium: 513mg. *Nutrition information is estimated and may vary depending on the ingredients used.

SALMON PASTA

Cook time: 20 minutes

Serving: 4

Ingredients:

- 1 lb dried pasta (any shape)
- 2 tbsp olive oil
- 4 cloves garlic, minced
- 1/4 tsp red pepper flakes (optional)
- 1/3 cup white wine or vegetable broth
- 2 skinless salmon fillets, cut into cubes (about 12 oz each)
- 2 lemons, juiced and zested
- 1/3 cup heavy cream
- 3/4 cup grated parmesan cheese
- Salt & pepper to taste

Preparation:

1. Bring a large pot of salted water to a boil over high heat. Add the pasta and cook according to package instructions until al dente. Drain and set aside.
2. In a large skillet, heat the olive oil over medium heat. Add the garlic and red pepper flakes (if using) and sauté for 1 minute, stirring often to prevent burning.
3. Add the white wine or broth and bring to a simmer. Add the salmon cubes and cook until just cooked through, about 3-4 minutes.

4. Add the lemon juice and zest, cream, parmesan cheese, salt & pepper to taste; stir well to combine all ingredients together in one saucepan over low heat for 2 minutes or until warmed through.

5. Serve warm over cooked pasta with extra Parmesan cheese, if desired.

Nutrition:

Calories: 590 Fat: 24g Carbohydrates: 58g Protein: 30g Sodium: 461mg Cholesterol: 89mg Fiber: 4g Sugar: 1.5g Vitamin A: 6% Vitamin C: 11% Calcium: 17% Iron: 8% Enjoy!

CRAB LEGS

Cook time: 20 minutes

Serving: 4 people

Ingredients:
- 2 pounds of crab legs
- 2 tablespoons of butter, melted
- 2 cloves garlic, minced
- 1 teaspoon Old Bay seasoning (or any other desired seasoning)
- Juice from half a lemon

Preparation:
1. Preheat the oven to 400°F (200°C). Line a baking sheet with parchment paper or aluminum foil.
2. Place the crab legs on the prepared baking sheet and brush them with melted butter. Sprinkle garlic and Old Bay seasoning over the top of the crab legs. Squeeze some fresh lemon juice over them as well.
3. Bake for about 15 minutes, or until the crab legs are cooked through and lightly golden.
4. Serve warm with additional lemon wedges, if desired.

Nutrition:

In a serving of two ounces (or approximately one small leg), there are approximately 85 calories, 1 gram of fat, 6 grams of protein and 398 milligrams of sodium. There is also trace amounts of calcium and iron. Enjoy!

CRUSTY PESTO SALMON

Cook time: 20 minutes

Serving: 4

Ingredients:

- 4 (6 ounce) salmon fillets
- 1/3 cup prepared basil pesto sauce
- 2 tablespoons grated Parmesan cheese
- Salt and freshly ground black pepper to taste
- 2 tablespoons olive oil, divided

Preparation:

1. Preheat oven to 375 degrees F (190 degrees C). Grease a baking sheet with 1 tablespoon of the olive oil.
2. Place salmon fillets onto baking sheet. Rub remaining olive oil over the top of each piece of salmon. Sprinkle Parmesan cheese on top of each fillet. Season with salt and pepper to taste.
3. Bake in preheated oven for 15 minutes, or until fish flakes easily with a fork.
4. Heat pesto sauce in a small skillet over medium heat. Once heated through, spoon pesto sauce over each salmon fillet.
5. Bake an additional 5 minutes, or until salmon is cooked through and the pesto sauce is bubbly. Serve immediately.

Nutrition:

Calories: 350 kcal; Protein: 31 g; Fat: 21 g; Cholesterol: 94 mg; Sodium 704 mg; Carbohydrates: 2 g; Fiber: 0g; Sugar: 0g.

BUTTERY COD

Cook Time: 2 minutes

Serving: 4 people

Ingredients:

- 2 tablespoons butter
- 4 cod fillets (approximately 5-6 ounces each)
- Salt and pepper to taste

Preparation:

1. Heat the butter in a large nonstick skillet over medium heat until melted and bubbly.
2. Place the cod fillets in the pan and season them with salt and pepper. Cook for 1 minute per side, or until the fish flakes easily with a fork.
3. Transfer the cod to a plate and serve.

Nutrition:

This buttery cod provides approximately 150 calories per serving, along with 15 grams of protein, 6 grams of fat, and 1 gram of carbohydrates. It is also a good source of omega3 fatty acids. Enjoy!

SESAME TUNA STEAK

Cook Time: 15 minutes

Servings: 4

Ingredients:

- 4 tuna steaks (1-inch thick)
- 2 tablespoons sesame oil
- 3 cloves of garlic, minced
- 1 teaspoon freshly grated ginger
- 2 tablespoons soy sauce
- 2 teaspoons brown sugar
- salt and pepper to taste

Preparation:

Heat the sesame oil in a large skillet over medium heat. Once hot, add the garlic and ginger, stirring for 1 minute until fragrant.

Add the tuna steaks and cook for 3 minutes per side or until golden and slightly charred.

Add the soy sauce, brown sugar, salt and pepper. Simmer until the sauce has slightly thickened.

Serve tuna steaks with the sesame-garlic sauce and enjoy!

Nutrition:

One serving of this sesame tuna steak contains 339 calories, 21g of fat, 16g of protein, 2g of carbohydrates, 1g of dietary fiber, and 1g of sugar. It also provides 17% of your recommended daily value (DV) for vitamin A and 20% DV for iron. Enjoy!

LEMON GARLIC SHRIMP

Cook time: 10 minutes

Servings: 4 people

Ingredients:

- 1 lb. shrimp, peeled and deveined
- 3 tablespoons extra-virgin olive oil
- 2 cloves garlic, minced
- Juice of 1 lemon
- Salt and pepper to taste

Preparation:

1. Heat the olive oil in a skillet over medium heat. Add the garlic and sauté for one minute or until fragrant.
2. Add the shrimp to the pan and season with salt and pepper. Cook for about 5 minutes, stirring occasionally, until the shrimp is just cooked through.
3. Remove from heat and add the lemon juice, stirring to combine.
4. Serve the shrimp with a side of your favorite vegetables or rice.

Nutrition:

One serving of this lemon garlic shrimp provides approximately 140 calories, 7 grams of fat, 1 gram of carbohydrates and 16 grams of protein. Additionally, it contains 0 grams of fiber, 2 mg cholesterol and about 300 mg sodium.

FOIL PACKET SALMON

Cook Time: 20 minutes

Servings: 4-6

Ingredients:

- 2 (7.5 oz) packets of salmon, thawed
- 4 tablespoons olive oil
- 1 teaspoon garlic powder
- 1/2 teaspoon black pepper
- Juice of 1 lemon
- Chopped parsley, to garnish (optional)

Preparation:

1. Preheat oven to 375°F. Grease a baking sheet with nonstick cooking spray and set aside.
2. Place the packets of salmon on the prepared baking sheet and brush each one with 2 tablespoons olive oil. Sprinkle with garlic powder and black pepper. Squeeze the juice of a lemon over each packet.
3. Bake for 15-20 minutes until salmon is cooked through and flakes easily with a fork.
4. Garnish with chopped parsley, if desired, and serve warm.

Nutrition:

Per Serving (calculated with 4 servings): 320 calories; 17g fat; 29g carbohydrate; 22g protein; 0mg cholesterol; 200mg sodium. Enjoy!

VEGETABLES

PARSLEY ZUCCHINI AND RADISHES

Cook Time: 10min

Servings: 4

Ingredients:

- 2 tablespoons olive oil
- 1 medium onion, chopped
- 3 cloves garlic, minced
- 1 large parsnip, peeled and chopped
- ½ cup celery, chopped
- 1 medium zucchini, diced
- 2-3 small radishes, thinly sliced
- ½ teaspoon oregano leaves
- ¼ teaspoon sea salt

Preparation:

1. Heat the oil in a large skillet or pot over medium heat. Add the onion and garlic and sauté for 5 minutes until the onions are soft.
2. Add the parsnip, celery, zucchini, and radishes and continue to cook for another 5 minutes.
3. Stir in the oregano leaves, sea salt, and pepper. Cook for an additional 2 minutes until all of the vegetables are tender.
4. Enjoy your parsley zucchini and radish dish!

Nutrition:

Per Serving (1/4 recipe): Calories 130; Total Fat 7g; Sodium 250mg; Total Carbohydrates 13g; Dietary Fiber 4g; Protein 2g.

CHERRY TOMATOES SAUTE

Cook Time: This cherry tomato sauté recipe takes just 10 minutes to prepare and cook!

Serving: This dish serves 4 people.

Ingredients:

- 2 tablespoons of olive oil
- 2 cloves of garlic, minced
- 2 pints of cherry tomatoes, halved or quartered
- 1/2 teaspoon of dried oregano
- Salt & pepper to taste

Preparation:

1. In a large skillet over medium-high heat, heat the olive oil until shimmering.
2. Add in the garlic and sauté for about one minute, stirring frequently.
3. Add in the cherry tomatoes and oregano and season with salt & pepper.
4. Reduce the heat to medium-low and cook, stirring occasionally, for 8-10 minutes until the tomatoes are softened.
5. Serve warm on its own or over grilled chicken or fish!

Nutrition:

One serving of this cherry tomato sauté recipe contains 108 calories, 7g of fat, 5g of carbohydrates, 7g of sugar, and 2g of protein. Additionally, it provides some minerals such as iron and folate at 1% each. This is a great option for a low-calorie side dish!

CREAMY EGGPLANT

Cook time: 20 minutes

Serving: 4-6 people

Ingredients:

- 1 large eggplant, diced
- 2 tablespoons olive oil
- Salt and freshly ground black pepper to taste
- 1/2 cup cream cheese
- 2 cloves garlic, minced
- 2 tablespoons chopped fresh basil leaves

Preparation:

1. Preheat the oven to 375 degrees F (190 degrees C). Grease a baking sheet with olive oil or line with parchment paper.
2. Place the diced eggplant onto the prepared baking sheet and drizzle with 2 tablespoons of olive oil; season generously with salt and pepper. Bake in preheated oven for 10 minutes, until tender but still firm.
3. In a small bowl, combine the cream cheese, garlic and basil.
4. Remove the eggplant from the oven and spread the cream cheese mixture over each piece of eggplant.
5. Return to the oven and bake for an additional 10 minutes until golden brown on top.
6. Serve warm with some fresh herbs or chopped tomatoes as garnish (optional).

Nutrition:

Each serving of creamy eggplant contains approximately 195 calories, 12 grams fat, 11 grams carbohydrates and 7 grams protein. It is also high in dietary fiber, vitamin A and iron. Additionally, it provides a good source of calcium and magnesium for healthy bones and teeth! Enjoy!

EGGPLANT AND CARROTS MIX

Cook Time: 15 minutes

Servings: 4

Ingredients:

- 3 cups eggplant, diced into 1/2-inch cubes
- 2 large carrots, diced into 1/4-inch cubes
- 2 tablespoons olive oil
- 1 teaspoon garlic powder
- Salt and pepper to taste

Preparation:

1. Preheat the oven to 350°F. Line a baking sheet with parchment paper.
2. Place the diced eggplant and carrots on the baking sheet and drizzle with olive oil. Sprinkle garlic powder, salt, and pepper on top of the vegetables. Gently toss everything together until evenly coated with oil and seasonings.
3. Bake in the preheated oven for 15 minutes, stirring halfway through. Serve warm or at room temperature.

Nutrition:

One serving of this vegetable mix provides 63 calories, 4 g fat, 6 g carbohydrates, and 2g protein. Additionally it is a source of dietary fiber and vitamin A. Enjoy!

PARMESAN EGGPLANTS

Cook Time: 15 minutes

Serving: 3-4 people

Ingredients:

- 2 small eggplants (cut into 1/2 inch slices)
- 1/2 cup olive oil
- 1/2 cup parmesan cheese (grated)
- Salt and pepper to taste

Preparation:

1. Preheat oven to 375 degrees F (190 degrees C). Place the sliced eggplant on a baking sheet lined with parchment paper or greased aluminum foil.
2. Drizzle olive oil over the eggplant slices and season with salt and pepper.
3. Bake in preheated oven for 10 minutes, or until lightly browned. Remove from oven and sprinkle parmesan cheese on top of the eggplant slices.
4. Return to oven for an additional 5 minutes, or until the parmesan cheese has melted. Serve warm and enjoy!

Nutrition:

Each serving of Parmesan Eggplants contains approximately 40 calories, 4 grams of fat, 1 gram of protein and 2 grams of carbohydrates. This dish is also a good source of vitamin C and iron. Enjoy!

KALE SAUTE

Cook Time: 10 minutes

Serving: 2 servings

Ingredients:

- 1 tablespoon olive oil
- 2 cloves garlic, minced
- 4 cups kale, finely chopped
- Salt and pepper to taste.

Preparation:

1. Heat the olive oil in a large skillet over medium heat. Add the garlic and cook for 1 minute until fragrant.
2. Add the kale to the skillet and stir occasionally for about 5 minutes until wilted. Season with salt and pepper to taste.
3. Serve warm on top of your favorite dish or as a side dish!

Nutrition Facts

(Per Serving): Calories 117, Total Fat 8g (Saturated fat 1g), Sodium 299mg, Carbohydrate 11g (Fiber 4g, Sugars 0.5g), Protein 5g. Calories from fat 69%.

CARROTS SAUTE

Cook Time: 10 minutes

Servings: 4

Ingredients:

- 2 tablespoons olive oil
- 1 tablespoon butter
- 2 cloves of garlic, minced
- 2 large carrots, peeled and sliced into discs
- Salt and pepper to taste

Preparation:

1. Heat the olive oil and butter in a large skillet over medium heat. Add the garlic and stir until fragrant, about 30 seconds.
2. Add the carrots to the pan and season with salt and pepper. Cook for 8 minutes or until they are tender, stirring occasionally.
3. Serve warm with your favorite side dish. Enjoy!

Nutrition Info :

(per serving): Calories: 90, Total Fat: 6g, Cholesterol: 10mg, Sodium: 150mg, Carbohydrates: 8g, Fiber: 2g, Sugars: 4g, Protein: 1g.

SPAGHETTI SQUASH CASSEROLE

Cook time: 30 minutes

Servings: 4

Ingredients:

- 1 medium spaghetti squash, cut in half lengthwise and seeded
- 2 tablespoons olive oil
- Salt and pepper to taste
- 1/4 cup grated Parmesan cheese
- 1/2 cup ricotta cheese

Preparation:

1. Preheat oven to 350 degrees F. Rub the inside of each squash half with olive oil and season with salt and pepper. Place the squash halves face down on a baking sheet lined with parchment paper or foil. Bake for 25 minutes until tender.

2. Remove from oven and allow to cool before handling it further. Once cooled, use a fork to scrape out the spaghetti-like strands from each squash half. Place the squash strands in a large bowl.

3. Add the Parmesan cheese, ricotta cheese and salt and pepper to taste. Stir until ingredients are combined thoroughly.

4. Lightly grease an 8x8 inch baking dish with olive oil or butter. Pour the squash mixture into it and spread evenly

with a spoon or rubber spatula. Top with extra Parmesan cheese if desired.

5. Bake for 25 minutes more until golden brown and heated through. Serve warm!

Nutrition:

One serving of Spaghetti Squash Casserole contains 190 calories, 9g fat, 18g carbohydrates, 7g protein, 2g fiber and 260mg sodium*.

SUPER TASTY ONION PETALS

Cook Time: 30 minutes

Servings: 4

Ingredients:

- 2 large sweet onions, sliced into thin petals
- 1 ½ cups all-purpose flour
- 1 teaspoon garlic powder
- 2 teaspoons smoked paprika
- 1 teaspoon salt
- 1 teaspoon freshly ground black pepper
- 2 ¼ cups light beer, divided (or sparkling water)
- Vegetable oil for frying

Preparation:

1. Place the sliced onion petals in a large bowl and set aside. In a separate bowl, combine the flour, garlic powder, smoked paprika, salt, and pepper. Slowly add in 1 cup of the beer or sparkling water until a thin batter forms.

2. Working in batches, dip the onion petals into the batter and coat evenly on all sides. Gently shake off any excess before transferring to a plate or sheet pan.

3. Heat about 2" of oil in a large pot over medium-high heat until it reaches 375°F (190°C). Line a separate plate with paper towels for draining the fried onions later.

4. Carefully drop several battered onion petals into the hot oil and fry until golden brown and crispy, 3-5 minutes per

batch. Transfer to the prepared plate lined with paper towels as they finish cooking to absorb any excess oil.

5. Serve warm with extra beer or sparkling water for dipping.

Nutrition Information:

(per serving): 250 calories, 13 g fat, 30 g carbohydrates, 4 g protein. Enjoy your freshly made onion petals!

EGGPLANT GARLIC SALAD WITH TOMATOES

Cook Time: 5 minutes

Servings: 4-6

Ingredients:

- 2 Eggplant (peeled and diced)
- 6 cloves Garlic (minced)
- 1 pint Cherry Tomatoes (halved)
- 2 tablespoons Olive Oil
- Salt & pepper (to taste)
- Parsley or Basil Leaves (optional, for garnish)

Preparation:

1. Preheat oven to 375°F/190°C. Place the eggplant on a baking sheet and roast in preheated oven for 10-15 minutes until soft and lightly browned. Allow to cool before proceeding with the recipe.
2. Heat olive oil in a large skillet over medium heat. Add garlic and cook for 1-2 minutes until fragrant.
3. Add eggplant to the skillet and season with salt and pepper to taste. Stir and cook for 3-4 minutes until eggplant is tender.
4. Add tomatoes to the skillet, stirring gently to combine. Cook for an additional 2-3 minutes until tomatoes are just beginning to soften.

5. Remove from heat and transfer Eggplant Garlic Salad into individual bowls or plates and garnish with parsley or basil leaves if desired. Serve warm or cool as desired!

Nutrition Information:

One serving of this Eggplant Garlic Salad provides approximately 166 calories, 12g fat, 9g carbohydrates, 5g protein and 6g dietary fiber. It is a good source of Vitamin C, Iron, Potassium and Manganese. Enjoy!

CURRY EGGPLANTS

Cook Time: 40 minutes

Serving: 4

Ingredients:

- 2 tablespoons vegetable oil
- 1 large onion, chopped
- 4 cloves garlic, minced
- 1 tablespoon ground cumin
- 1 tablespoon ground coriander
- 2 teaspoons ground turmeric
- 1/2 teaspoon chili powder (optional)
- 2 medium-sized eggplants, cut into cubes
- 2 tomatoes, chopped
- 1/2 teaspoon salt, or to taste

Preparation:

1. Heat oil in a large skillet over medium heat. Add the onion and garlic, and cook until softened and lightly browned, about 5 minutes.
2. Add cumin, coriander, turmeric, chili powder (if using), eggplant cubes and tomatoes to the skillet. Stir to combine all ingredients together.
3. Reduce heat to low and simmer for 25-30 minutes or until the eggplant is tender.

4. Season with salt (to taste) at the end of cooking time and serve hot with basmati rice or roti/naan bread!

Nutrition:

Curry Eggplants is rich in fiber, vitamins A & C, potassium as well as other essential nutrients. It also contains healthy fats from the vegetable oil used to prepare it and is low in calories! One serving of Curry Eggplants provides approximately 150-200 calories. Enjoy!

SAUTEED ASPARAGUS

Cook time: 10-15 minutes

Servings: 4

Ingredients:

- 1 pound asparagus, ends trimmed
- 2 tablespoons olive oil
- 2 cloves garlic, minced
- Salt and pepper to taste

Preparation:

1. Preheat oven to 400 degrees F (200 degrees C). Place the asparagus on a baking sheet.
2. Drizzle with olive oil and sprinkle with garlic, salt and pepper. Toss lightly to combine.
3. Bake in preheated oven for 10 to 15 minutes, or until the asparagus is tender when pierced with a fork. Remove from heat and serve immediately.

Nutrition:

Calories: 66; Total Fat: 4.8g; Saturated Fat: 0.6g; Cholesterol: 0mg; Sodium: 10mg ; Carbohydrates: 5.5g ; Protein: 2.7g ; Fiber : 1.9g ; Sugar : 1.9 g. Enjoy! :-)

ROASTED APPLE WITH BACON

Cook Time: 25 minutes

Servings: 4 servings

Ingredients:

- 2 apples, peeled and cored
- 1 tablespoon butter
- 4 slices bacon, cooked and chopped
- ¼ teaspoon ground cinnamon
- 1 tablespoon brown sugar

Preparation:

1. Preheat oven to 350°F (176°C). Grease a baking dish with some butter or cooking spray.
2. Place the peeled and cored apples in the prepared baking dish. Dot each apple with some of the butter.
3. Sprinkle with cinnamon and brown sugar, then top with chopped bacon pieces.
4. Bake for 20-25 minutes, or until apples are tender. Serve warm.

Nutrition:

Calories: 144, Fat: 5g, Saturated Fat: 2.3g, Cholesterol: 14mg, Sodium: 112mg, Potassium: 167mg, Carbohydrates: 24g, Fiber: 4g, Sugar: 15g, Protein: 2.6g. Enjoy!

FENNEL SLICES

Cook Time: 15 minutes

Servings: 4-6

Ingredients:

- 2 medium fennel bulbs, thinly sliced
- 1 tablespoon olive oil
- Salt and pepper to taste

Preparation:

1. Preheat oven to 375°F (190°C). Grease a baking sheet with nonstick cooking spray or line it with parchment paper.
2. Slice the bulbs into thin slices and toss them in a bowl with the olive oil, salt, and pepper.
3. Spread the slices onto the prepared baking sheet in an even layer and bake for 10-15 minutes or until golden brown. Serve warm or at room temperature.

Nutrition Information

(per serving): Calories: 70 Fat: 4g Carbohydrates: 8g Protein: 1.5g Fiber: 2.5g Sugar: 1g Sodium: 150mg Cholesterol: 0mg. Enjoy!

BUTTERNUT SQUASH RICE

Cook Time: 25 minutes

Servings: 4

Ingredients:

- 1 butternut squash, peeled and cubed
- 2 tablespoons olive oil
- Salt and pepper to taste
- 1 cup uncooked long-grain white rice
- 4 cups vegetable broth

Preparation:

1. Preheat the oven to 400°F (200°C). Place the cubed butternut squash onto a baking sheet lined with parchment paper. Drizzle with olive oil, salt, and pepper and mix until evenly coated. Roast in the preheated oven for 20-25 minutes or until softened. Set aside.
2. In a medium pot over medium heat, bring the vegetable broth to a boil. Add the rice, reduce the heat to low and simmer for 18-20 minutes, stirring occasionally.
3. When the rice is cooked, stir in the roasted butternut squash and mix until combined. Serve warm.

Nutrition:

Butternut squash is a great source of dietary fiber, vitamin C, potassium and magnesium. This dish provides about 4 grams of dietary fiber per serving. Enjoy!

EGGPLANT LASAGNA

Cook time: 45 minutes

Serving: 6-8 people

Ingredients:

- 2 large eggplants, cut into ¼ inch slices
- 1 teaspoon of salt
- 4 tablespoons of olive oil
- 2 cloves garlic, minced
- 1 28 oz can of crushed tomatoes
- 8 ounces of lasagna noodles
- 3 cups ricotta cheese
- 1 cup shredded mozzarella cheese

Preparation:

1. Preheat oven to 375 degrees F (190 degrees C). Grease a 9x13 inch baking dish.
2. Place the sliced eggplant in a single layer on a baking sheet. Sprinkle with salt and drizzle with 2 tablespoons of olive oil. Bake for 15 minutes, turning once after about 7 minutes. Remove from oven and set aside.
3. Heat remaining 2 tablespoons of olive oil in a large skillet over medium heat. Add garlic, and cook until fragrant, about 1 minute. Pour in the crushed tomatoes and bring to a simmer. Simmer for 10 minutes.
4. Place 4 lasagna noodles in the bottom of the prepared baking dish, overlapping as necessary to fit them all into

one layer. Spread approximately ½ cup of ricotta cheese evenly over the noodles, followed by ½ cup of mozzarella cheese, then spread 1/3 of the cooked tomato sauce over top. Layer on half of the eggplant slices, followed by another layer of lasagna noodles, ricotta cheese, mozzarella cheese and tomato sauce. Top with remaining eggplant slices and finish with a final layer of noodles, ricotta cheese, mozzarella cheese and tomato sauce.

5. Cover baking dish with foil and bake for 30 minutes. Remove foil and continue baking for an additional 15 minutes until top is lightly golden browned and bubbling around the edges. Let stand for 10 minutes before serving.

Nutrition:

Calories: 402; Total Fat: 20g; Saturated Fat: 9g; Cholesterol: 40mg; Sodium : 883mg; Carbohydrates: 36g; Fiber: 7.6g; Sugar: 9.4g; Protein: 19.3g.

STUFFED EGGPLANTS WITH CHERRY TOMATOES

Cook Time: The total cook time for this recipe is about 25 minutes.

Serving: This recipe will make four servings.

Ingredients:

- 4 small-medium eggplants
- 1/2 cup diced red onion
- 2 tablespoons olive oil
- 2 cloves garlic, minced
- 2 cups cherry tomatoes, halved
- 1/4 cup fresh basil leaves, chopped
- 3 tablespoons balsamic vinegar
- Salt and pepper to taste

Preparation:

- Preheat the oven to 350 degrees F. Slice the eggplants in half lengthwise and scoop out the centers. Drizzle the olive oil into a large skillet over medium heat, add the diced onion, and sauté until tender. Add the garlic and cook for another minute or two.

- Add the halved cherry tomatoes to the pan and simmer for about five minutes until they begin to soften. Add salt and pepper to taste. Remove from heat, stir in chopped basil leaves, and set aside.

- Place each eggplant half on a baking sheet lined with parchment paper; spoon tomato mixture into each one evenly. Drizzle each stuffed eggplant with balsamic vinegar then bake at 350°F for 15-20 minutes. Serve warm.

Nutrition:

Each serving of the stuffed eggplant with cherry tomatoes contains about 132 calories, 7 g fat, 16 g carbohydrates, and 4 g protein. This recipe is also an excellent source of dietary fiber and vitamins A, C, and K. Enjoy!

SALADS

SATISFYING SPRING SALAD

Cook Time: 10 minutes

Servings: 4

Ingredients:

- 3 cups of baby spinach leaves, washed and dried
- 1/2 cup red onion, diced small
- 1/2 cup sliced mushrooms
- 1/4 cup crumbled feta cheese
- 1 tsp garlic powder
- 2 tbsp olive oil
- 1 lemon (juiced)
- Salt & pepper to taste

Preparation Instructions:

1. Preheat oven to 375°F. Place the spinach leaves in a large bowl. In a separate bowl, combine the diced red onion, mushrooms, feta cheese, garlic powder and olive oil. Mix together until everything is well combined.
2. Pour the mixture over the spinach leaves and toss to coat evenly. Squeeze the lemon juice on top and season with salt & pepper to taste.
3. Place salad onto a baking sheet lined with parchment paper and cook for 10 minutes or until vegetables are tender.
4. Serve warm or cold, as desired! Enjoy!

Nutrition Facts:

(per serving): Calories: 115 Fat: 8g Carbohydrates: 7g Protein: 4g Fiber: 2g Sodium: 123mg Cholesterol: 8mg.

THE RAW GREEN DETOX SALAD

Cook Time: 10 minutes

Serving: 3-4 People

Ingredients:

- 2 cups of spinach
- 1/2 cup of broccoli florets
- 1 small avocado, diced
- 1/4 cup cucumber, diced
- 1/2 cup cherry tomatoes, halved
- 1/4 cup fresh parsley, chopped
- 2 tablespoons olive oil
- Juice from half a lemon

Preparation:

1. In a large bowl, combine spinach and broccoli. Toss to combine.
2. Add in the avocado, cucumber, tomatoes and parsley. Toss together to combine.
3. Drizzle the olive oil and lemon juice over the salad and toss to coat.
4. Serve chilled or at room temperature.

Nutrition Facts:

Calories: 220 Total Fat: 17g

Saturated Fat: 3g Cholesterol: 0mg Sodium: 32mg

Carbohydrates: 12g Fiber: 4g Protein: 6g

DANDELION SALAD

Cook Time: 10 minutes

Servings: 4

Ingredients:

- 2 bunches of dandelion greens, washed and roughly chopped
- 1/4 cup olive oil
- 1/4 cup white wine vinegar or apple cider vinegar
- 2 cloves garlic, minced
- Salt and pepper to taste

Preparation:

1. Heat the olive oil in a large skillet over medium heat. Add the garlic and sauté for 1-2 minutes.
2. Add the dandelion greens to the pan and season with salt and pepper. Cook for 3-4 minutes, stirring occasionally, until the leaves are wilted.
3. In a small bowl whisk together the vinegar and olive oil until combined.
4. Pour the dressing over the dandelion greens and stir to combine. Serve immediately.

Nutrition:

Calories: 114kcal Carbohydrates: 4g Protein: 2g Fat: 10g Saturated Fat: 1g Sodium: 60mg Potassium: 332mg Fiber: 1g Sugar: 1g Vitamin A: 5192IU Vitamin C: 29mg Calcium: 116mg Iron 2mg.

SPICY WAKAME SALAD

Cook Time: 10 Minutes

Serving: 2 people

Ingredients:

- 2 cups of Wakame seaweed, soaked and drained
- 1 teaspoon of sesame oil
- 1 tablespoon of soy sauce
- 1 tablespoon of rice vinegar
- 2 tablespoons of chili oil or pepper flakes

Preparation:

1. In a medium bowl, combine the wakame seaweed, sesame oil, soy sauce and rice vinegar. Mix well until all ingredients are evenly distributed.
2. Heat a large skillet over medium heat for about one minute and add the chili oil or pepper flakes to the pan. Add the prepared wakame salad mix from step one and sauté for 3-5 minutes.
3. Plate the spicy wakame salad and enjoy!

Nutrition:

Per serving: 54 Calories, 2g Fat, 4g Carbohydrates, 0g Protein. This is a low calorie delicious vegan side dish that can be enjoyed as part of any meal! Enjoy!

AVO-ORANGE SALAD DISH

Cook Time: 10 minutes

Serving: 4

Ingredients:

- 2 avocados, diced
- 3 oranges, peeled and cut into cubes
- 1/3 cup walnuts, chopped
- 2 tablespoons olive oil
- Juice from one lime
- Salt and pepper to taste

Preparation:

1. In a medium bowl, combine all ingredients until mixed together.
2. Serve immediately with extra lime juice, if desired.

Nutrition

Per Serving: (1/4 of recipe) Calories – 177, Fat – 11.6g, Carbohydrates – 13.8g, Protein – 2.7g.

NOURISHING ELECTRIC SALAD

Cook Time: 10 minutes

Serving: 4-6 people

Ingredients:

- 1 cup of kale, chopped
- ½ cup quinoa, cooked and cooled
- 1 red bell pepper, diced
- ½ cucumber, diced
- ¼ cup freshly minced parsley
- 2 tablespoons olive oil
- 2 tablespoons lemon juice
- Salt and pepper to taste

Preparation:

1. In a large bowl, combine the kale, quinoa, bell pepper, cucumber and parsley.
2. Drizzle with olive oil and lemon juice then season with salt and pepper to taste. Mix everything together until well combined.
3. Serve the salad immediately or chill it in the refrigerator for 1-2 hours before serving.

Nutrition:

One serving of this Nourishing Electric Salad contains approximately 150 calories, 7 g fat, 16 g carbohydrates and 4 g protein. It also provides generous amounts of vitamins A and C, iron, magnesium and dietary fiber. Enjoy!

SUPERFOOD FONIO SALAD

Cook time: 15 minutes

Servings: 4-6 people

Ingredients:

- 2 cups of fonio grains
- 2 tablespoons olive oil
- 1/4 cup diced red onion
- 1 cup chopped cucumber
- 1/2 cup cherry tomatoes, quartered
- 1/3 cup crumbled feta cheese
- Salt and pepper to taste

Preparation:

1. In a medium saucepan, bring three cups of water to a boil over medium heat. Once boiling, add one cup of fonio and reduce the heat to low. Simmer for 10-12 minutes or until the fonio is cooked through and soft. Drain the fonio, rinse with cold water and set aside.

2. Heat olive oil in a large skillet over medium heat. Add the red onion and sauté for 3-4 minutes or until tender.

3. Add the cucumber, fonio and tomatoes to the pan, stirring to combine everything together. Cook for another 5 minutes, stirring occasionally.

4. Remove from heat and stir in feta cheese, salt and pepper to taste. Serve warm or cold!

Nutrition:

Each serving contains approximately 200 calories with 9 grams of protein, 24 grams of carbohydrates and 11 grams of fat. Fonio is also a great source of fiber providing 4% of your daily needs per serving! Enjoy!

HEALTHY CHICKPEA ROAST SALAD

Cook Time: 25 minutes

Servings: 4-6 people

Ingredients:
- 2 cans of chickpeas, drained and rinsed
- 1 red bell pepper, diced
- 2 tablespoons of olive oil
- Salt and pepper to taste
- 1 teaspoon of garlic powder
- ½ teaspoon of chili flakes (optional)

Preparation:
1. Preheat your oven to 375F/ 190C.
2. In a large bowl, mix together the chickpeas, red bell pepper, olive oil, salt and pepper and garlic powder until everything is evenly coated.
3. Spread out the mixture on a lined baking tray. Roast in the oven for 20-25 minutes, or until lightly browned and crispy.
4. Serve warm with a sprinkle of chili flakes (optional). Enjoy!

Nutrition Facts:

Calories: 320kcal Protein: 9.5g Carbohydrates: 36g

Fat: 14g Fiber: 8.7g

AMARANTH TABBOULEH SALAD

Cook Time: 10 minutes

Servings: 6-8

Ingredients:

- 1 cup uncooked amaranth grains
- 2 cups vegetable broth or water
- 3/4 cup cooked bulgur wheat
- 2 tablespoons olive oil
- 1 small onion, diced
- 2 cloves garlic, minced
- 1 large tomato, chopped
- 1/3 cucumber, peeled and diced
- 2 tablespoons freshly squeezed lemon juice
- 2 tablespoons fresh parsley, chopped
- Salt and pepper to taste

Preparation:

1. Heat the olive oil in a medium saucepan over medium heat. Add the onion and garlic and sauté until the onion is soft, about 5 minutes.

2. Add the amaranth and stir to coat with the oil and vegetables. Then add the vegetable broth or water and bring to a boil. Reduce heat to low, cover, and simmer until all of the liquid is absorbed, 10-15 minutes. Remove from heat and let cool for 10 minutes before adding other ingredients.

3. In a large bowl combine cooked amaranth with bulgur wheat, tomato, cucumber, lemon juice, parsley, salt and pepper to taste; mix well.

4. Serve warm or chilled as a side dish or main course salad. Enjoy!

Nutrition:

Amaranth tabbouleh salad is a nutritious and flavorful dish. Each serving provides 4 grams of protein, 8 grams of dietary fiber, 10% Vitamin A (from the tomato), 15% Vitamin C (from the lemon juice), and 25% calcium (from the amaranth). Enjoy!

ZUCCHINI AND MUSHROOM BOWL

Cook time: 10 minutes

Serving: 4 servings

Ingredients:

- 1 cup cooked quinoa
- 1 small zucchini, cut into thin strips
- 2 large mushrooms, sliced
- 2 tablespoons olive oil
- 1 teaspoon garlic powder
- Salt and pepper to taste

Preparation:

1. In a medium bowl, combine cooked quinoa, zucchini strips, mushrooms, olive oil, and garlic powder. Season with salt and pepper to taste. Mix well until all ingredients are evenly distributed.
2. Heat a large skillet over medium heat. Add the quinoa-vegetable mixture and cook for 810 minutes or until vegetables start to soften.
3. Serve in individual bowls and enjoy!

Nutrition Information:

One serving contains approximately 150 calories, 9 grams of fat, 14 grams of carbohydrates, and 4 grams of protein.

QUINOA, TOMATO, AND MANGO SALAD

Cook Time: 15 minutes

Servings: 4

Ingredients:

- 1 cup uncooked quinoa
- 2 cups water
- ½ teaspoon salt
- 1 tablespoon olive oil
- 1 cup cherry tomatoes, halved
- ½ cup diced red onion
- ¼ cup sliced almonds
- ½ cup diced mangoes
- 2 tablespoons lemon juice
- 2 tablespoons chopped fresh parsley

Preparation:

1. In a medium saucepan, bring the quinoa, water, and salt to a boil over medium-high heat. Reduce the heat to low and simmer for 12 minutes, or until the quinoa is tender. Remove from the heat and set aside.

2. Heat the olive oil in a large skillet over medium-high heat. Add in the tomatoes, onion, almonds and mangoes and cook for 4-5 minutes or until everything is softened and lightly browned.

3. Add in the cooked quinoa to the pan and stir to combine with all of the other ingredients before adding in lemon juice and parsley. Stir one more time and remove from heat.

4. Serve warm or cold. Enjoy!

Nutrition:

Per serving, this quinoa salad contains 229 calories, 11 grams of fat, 4 grams of protein, 28 grams of carbohydrates, and 5 grams of dietary fiber. It is a great source of vitamins A and C as well as iron and calcium.

www.ingramcontent.com/pod-product-compliance
Lightning Source LLC
Chambersburg PA
CBHW071451080526
44587CB00014B/2065